Pocket Guide to
Basic Dysrhythmias

Interpretation and Management

ROBERT J. HUSZAR, MD
Former Medical Director, Emergency Medical Services
New York State Department of Health, Albany, New York

REVISED THIRD EDITION
*with **122** illlustrations*

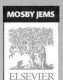

MOSBY JEMS

ELSEVIER

D1536936

MOSBY JEMS
ELSEVIER

11830 Westline Industrial Drive
St. Louis, Missouri 63146

Pocket Guide to Basic Dysrhythmias: Interpretation and Management
Revised Third Edition

NOTICE
Knowledge and best practice in this field are constantly changing. As new research and experience broaden our knowledge, changes in practice, treatment and drug therapy may become necessary or appropriate. Readers are advised to check the most current information provided (i) on procedures featured or (ii) by the manufacturer of each product to be administered, to verify the recommended dose or formula, the method and duration of administration, and contraindications. It is the responsibility of the practitioner, relying on their own experience and knowledge of the patient, to make diagnoses, to determine dosages and the best treatment for each individual patient, and to take all appropriate safety precautions. To the fullest extent of the law, neither the Publisher nor the Editor assume any liability for any injury and/or damage to persons or property arising out or related to any use of the material contained in this book.

ISBN-13: 978-0-323-04857-6
ISBN-10: 0-323-04857-9
Publishing Director: Andrew Allen
Executive Editor: Linda Honeycutt
Developmental Editor: Katherine Tomber
Publishing Services Manager: John Rogers
Design Direction: Teresa McBryan, Kimberly Denando

Printed in the United States of America

Last digit is the print number: 9 8 7 6 5 4 3 2 1

This book is dedicated to my wife,

Jean

PREFACE

The **Pocket Guide to Basic Dysrhythmias** is intended to be used as a pocket reference in the interpretation of arrhythmias, bundle branch and fascicular blocks, miscellaneous electrocardiogram (ECG) changes (such as occur in chamber enlargement, pericarditis, electrolyte imbalance, drug administration, pulmonary disease, early repolarization, hypothermia, and preexcitation syndromes), and ECG patterns in acute myocardial infarction (MI). The interpretation of arrhythmias and some of the miscellaneous ECG changes rely on the analysis of a single ECG lead, usually lead II, whereas the identification of bundle branch and fascicular blocks, acute MI, and the rest of the miscellaneous ECG changes rely on the analysis of the 12-lead ECG.

The pocket guide also includes basic information on the electrical conduction system of the heart and its coronary circulation; the placement of leads in monitoring ECG leads I, II, III, MCL_1, and MCL_6 and a 12-lead ECG; the derivation of the hexaxial reference figure, the lead axes and their perpendiculars, and the normal and abnormal QRS axes; the three-lead method of determining the QRS axis; the components of the ECG; and the steps in interpreting the ECG and the methods of determining the heart rate.

Finally, the pocket guide includes sections on the treatment of arrhythmias and acute MI, which reflect the findings of:

- 2005 American Heart Association Guidelines for Cardiopulmonary Resuscitation and Emergency Cardiovascular Care
- Krumholz HM et al: ACC/AHA Clinical Performance Measures for Adults With ST-Elevation and Non-ST-Elevation Myocardial Infarction: a Report of the American College of Cardiology/American Heart Association Task Force on Performance Measures (Writing Committee to Develop Performance Measures on ST-Elevation and Non-ST-Elevation Myocardial Infarction), *J Am Coll Cardiol* 47:236-265, 2006 (2006 update available at *www.acc.org*).
- Ryan TJ et al: ACC/AHA guidelines for the management of patients with acute myocardial infarction: a report of the American College of Cardiology/American Heart Association Task Force on Practice Guidelines (Committee on Management of Acute Myocardial Infarction), *J Am Coll Cardiol* 28:1328-1428, 1996 (1999 update available at *www.acc.org*).

The **Pocket Guide to Basic Dysrhythmias** is also intended to complement **Basic Dysrhythmias,** revised third edition, from which the text, illustrations, and ECGs were abstracted and then modified to some extent by the author.

A NOTE TO THE READER

The author and publisher have made every attempt to check dosages and advanced life support content for accuracy. The care procedures presented here represent accepted practices in the United States. They are not offered as a standard of care. Advanced life support level emergency care is performed under the authority of a licensed physician. It is the reader's responsibility to know and follow local care protocols as provided by his or her medical advisers. It is also the reader's responsibility to stay informed of emergency care procedure changes, including the most recent guidelines set forth by the American Heart Association and printed in their textbooks.

I would like to acknowledge the following reviewers for their work on this edition: *Robert Cook,* EMT-P, EMD, I/C, Paramedic Supervisor, Hamilton Hospital, Webster City, Iowa; and *Robert Carter,* NREMT-P, Instructor, Baltimore City Fire Department Faculty, Hopkins Outreach for Pediatric Education, The Johns Hopkins Children's Center, Baltimore.

Robert J. Huszar

CONTENTS

Appendix, 131

SECTION

Arrhythmia Identification

NORMAL SINUS RHYTHM (NSR)

Heart Rate: 60-100/min.

Rhythm: Essentially regular.

Pacemaker Site: SA node.

P Waves: Upright in lead II; identical and precede each QRS complex.

PR Intervals: Normal (0.12-0.20 sec); constant.

R-R Intervals: Equal.

QRS Complexes: Usually normal (0.10 sec or less), unless a preexisting intraventricular conduction disturbance* is present.

Treatment: None.

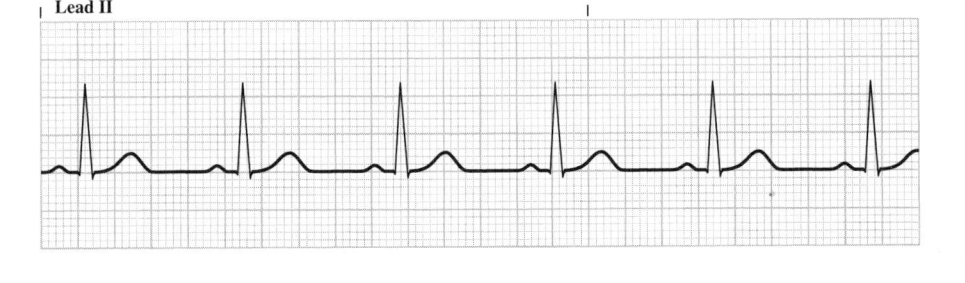

Lead II

---

*The most common form of intraventricular conduction disturbance is a right or left bundle branch block. A less common form is a nonspecific, diffuse intraventricular conduction defect (IVCD) seen in myocardial infarction (MI), fibrosis, and hypertrophy; electrolyte imbalance, such as hypokalemia and hyperkalemia; and excessive administration of such cardiac drugs as quinidine and procainamide.

SINUS ARRHYTHMIA

Heart Rate: 60-100/min. Typically, the heart rate increases during inspiration and decreases during expiration.

Rhythm: Regularly irregular.

Pacemaker Site: SA node.

P Waves: Upright in lead II: identical and precede each QRS complex.

PR Intervals: Normal (0.12-0.20 sec); constant.

R-R Intervals: Unequal; shorter during inspiration, longer during expiration.

QRS Complexes: Usually normal (0.10 sec or less), unless a preexisting intraventricular conduction disturbance is present.

Treatment: None.

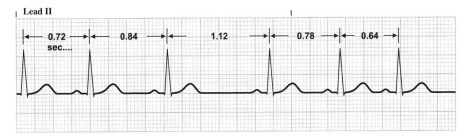

SINUS BRADYCARDIA

Heart Rate: Less than 60/min.

Rhythm: Essentially regular.

Pacemaker Site: SA node.

P Waves: Upright in lead II; identical and precede each QRS complex.

PR Intervals: Normal (0.12-0.20 sec); constant.

R-R Intervals: Equal.

QRS Complexes: Usually normal (0.10 sec or less), unless a preexisting intraventricular conduction disturbance is present.

Treatment: See Section II, page 36.

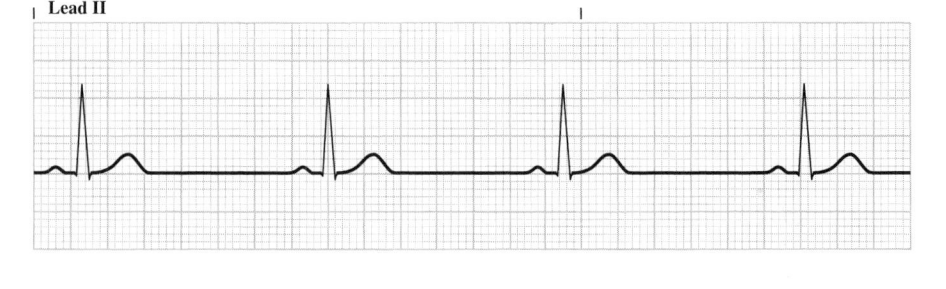

Lead II

SINUS ARREST AND SINOATRIAL (SA) EXIT BLOCK

Heart Rate: 60-100/min or less.

Rhythm: Irregular when sinus arrest or SA exit block is present.

Pacemaker Site: SA node.

P Waves: Absent when sinus arrest or SA exit block is present (dropped P wave).

PR Intervals: Absent when sinus arrest or SA exit block is present.

R-R Intervals: Unequal when sinus arrest or SA exit block is present.

QRS Complexes: Usually normal (0.10 sec or less), unless a preexisting intraventricular conduction disturbance is present.

Treatment: See Section II, page 36.

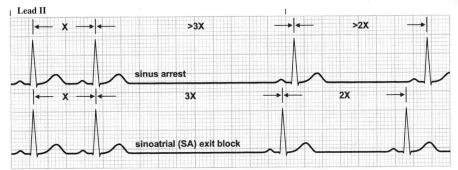

Lead II

X | >3X | >2X
sinus arrest

X | 3X | 2X
sinoatrial (SA) exit block

SINUS TACHYCARDIA

Heart Rate: Greater than 100/min, can be as high as 180/min or greater.

Rhythm: Essentially regular.

Pacemaker Site: SA node.

P Waves: Normal, or slightly taller and more peaked than normal; upright in lead II; identical and precede each QRS complex.

PR Intervals: Normal (0.12-0.20 sec); constant.

R-R Intervals: Usually equal, but may be slightly unequal.

QRS Complexes: Usually normal (0.10 sec or less), unless a preexisting intraventricular conduction disturbance or aberrant ventricular conduction* is present.

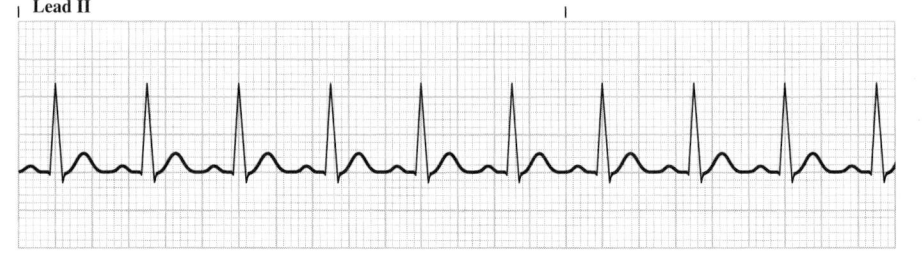

Lead II

Treatment: No specific treatment indicated. See Section II, page 38.

---

*A temporary delay in the conduction of an electrical impulse through the bundle branches producing an abnormally wide QRS complex, caused by the appearance of the electrical impulse at the bundle branches prematurely while they are still partially refractory and unable to conduct normally. The QRS complex may show a right or left bundle branch block pattern or a combination of a right bundle branch block pattern and a left anterior or posterior fascicular block pattern.

WANDERING ATRIAL PACEMAKER (WAP)

Heart Rate: Usually 60-100/min, but may be less.

Rhythm: Usually irregular.

Pacemaker Site: Shifts back and forth between the SA node and an ectopic pacemaker in the atria or atrioventricular (AV) junction.

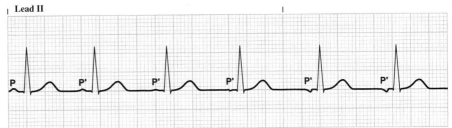

P Waves: Gradually change in size, shape, and direction from normal, positive (upright) P waves to abnormally small, even negative (inverted) P' waves over a series of beats, and then back again to normal in a reverse sequence; precede each QRS complex.

PR Intervals: Unequal; varies within normal limits (0.12-0.20 sec) from about 0.20 sec to about 0.12 sec over a series of beats and then back again.

R-R Intervals: Usually unequal.

QRS Complexes: Usually normal (0.10 sec or less), unless a preexisting intraventricular conduction disturbance is present.

Treatment: No specific treatment indicated.

PREMATURE ATRIAL CONTRACTIONS (PACs)

Heart Rate: That of the underlying rhythm.

Rhythm: Irregular when PACs are present.

Pacemaker Site: An ectopic pacemaker in the atria.

P′ Waves: P′ waves occur earlier than the next expected P wave of the underlying rhythm. They vary in size, shape, and direction in any given lead depending on the site of their origin,

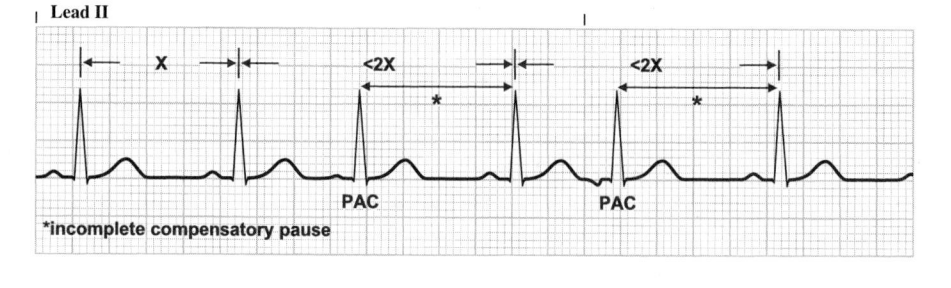

being positive (upright) in lead II if the pacemaker site is near the SA node or negative (inverted) if the pacemaker site is near the AV junction. P′ waves followed by QRS complexes related to them are *conducted PACs*. P′ waves occurring alone, not followed by QRS complexes, are *nonconducted, dropped,* or *blocked PACs*.

P-P Intervals: The P-P′ interval (coupling interval) is usually shorter, and the P′-P interval is the same or slightly longer than the P-P interval of the underlying rhythm. Commonly, an incomplete compensatory pause is present (i.e., the sum of the P-P′ and the P′-P intervals is less than twice the P-P interval of the underlying rhythm). Rarely, a com-

plete compensatory pause is present (i.e., the sum of the P-P′ and the P′-P intervals is equal to twice the underlying P-P interval).

P′R Intervals: Normal (0.12-0.20 sec); may vary between PACs.

R-R Intervals: Unequal when PACs are present.

QRS Complexes: Usually normal (0.10 sec or less), resembling those of the underlying rhythm. If aberrant ventricular conduction is present, the PAC may be wide and bizarre, resembling a PVC—PAC with aberrancy.

Treatment: See Section II, page 57.

TYPES OF PACs

Infrequent PACs: Less than five PACs/min.

Frequent PACs: Five or more PACs/min.

Isolated PACs (Beats): PACs occurring singly.

Group Beats: PACs occurring in groups of two or more.

Paired PACs (Couplet): Two PACs in a row.

Atrial Tachycardia: Three or more PACs in a row.

Atrial Bigeminy: PACs alternating with the QRS complexes of the underlying rhythm.

Atrial Trigeminy/Atrial Quadrigeminy: PACs following every two or three QRS complexes of the underlying rhythm, respectively.

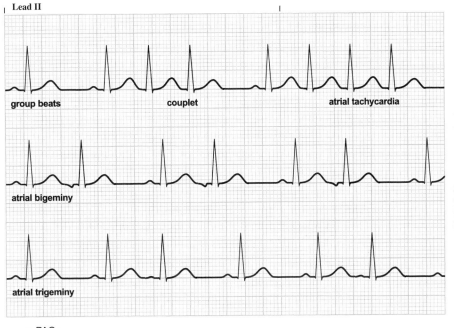

Lead II

group beats   couplet   atrial tachycardia

atrial bigeminy

atrial trigeminy

— = PACs

ATRIAL TACHYCARDIA
(ECTOPIC ATRIAL TACHYCARDIA, MULTIFOCAL ATRIAL TACHYCARDIA [MAT])

Heart Rate: Usually 160-240/min.

Rhythm: Essentially regular. Onset and termination are usually gradual.

Pacemaker Site: An ectopic pacemaker in the atria. When a single ectopic pacemaker site is present, the arrhythmia is called *ectopic atrial tachycardia;* when three or more pacemaker sites are present, it is called *multifocal atrial tachycardia (MAT).*

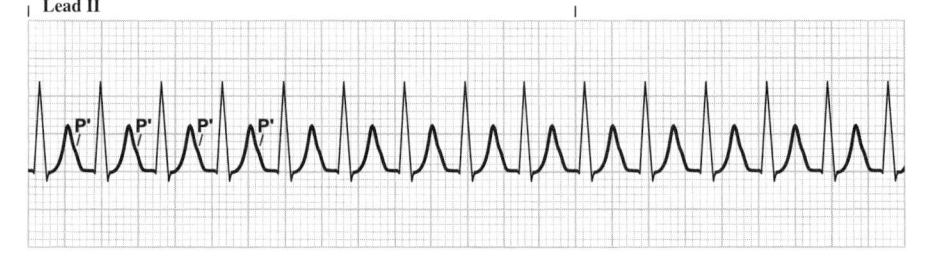

Lead II

P′ Waves: The P′ waves, which usually precede the QRS complexes, may be either: (1) positive (upright) in lead II if they originate in the atria near the SA node or (2) negative (inverted) if they originate in the atria near the AV junction. The P′ waves are usually identical in any given lead in ectopic atrial tachycardia, but in MAT they vary in size, shape, and direction in each given lead. When P′ waves are not always followed by a QRS complex, atrial tachycardia with block is present (e.g., a 2:1, 3:1, or 4:1 block). The P′ waves are often buried in the preceding T or U waves or QRS complexes.

P′R Intervals: The P′R intervals are usually normal (0.12-0.20 sec) and constant in ectopic atrial tachycardia; in MAT they vary slightly from 0.20 sec to less than 0.12 sec in each given lead.

R-R Intervals: Usually equal in ectopic atrial tachycardia without block, but will vary in MAT. The R-R intervals will also vary in atrial tachycardia with block.

QRS Complexes: Usually normal (0.10 sec or less), unless a preexisting intraventricular conduction disturbance, aberrant ventricular conduction, or ventricular preexcitation* is present. If the wide and bizarre QRS complexes occur only with the atrial tachycardia, the arrhythmia is called *atrial tachycardia with aberrancy* (or *atrial tachycardia with aberrant ventricular conduction).* Such a tachycardia usually resembles ventricular tachycardia.

Treatment: See Section II, pages 39 and 41.

---

*Abnormal conduction of electrical impulses from the atria to the ventricles via an accessory AV pathway bypassing the AV junction and causing premature activation of the ventricles. This commonly results in a shorter than normal PR interval (0.09-0.12 sec) and a wide QRS complex (greater than 0.10 sec) with an initial slurring of the upward slope of the R wave (the delta wave).

ATRIAL FLUTTER

Heart Rate: *Atrial rate:* 240-360 (average, 300) F waves/min. *Ventricular rate:* Usually about 150/min if atrial flutter is uncontrolled (untreated); 60-75/min if controlled (treated) or if a preexisting AV block is present.

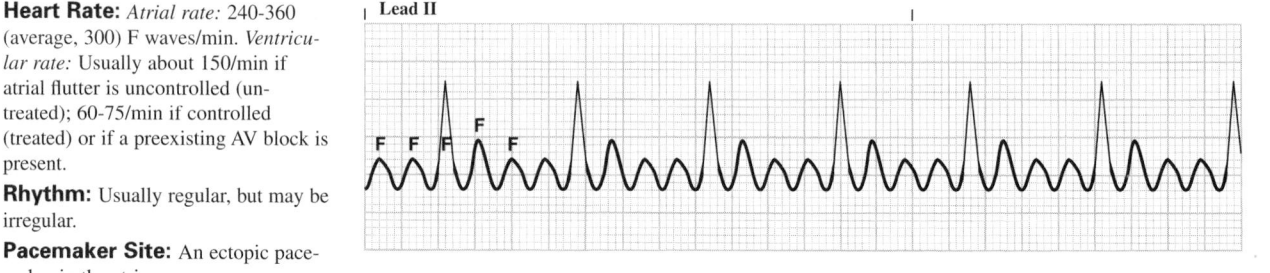

Rhythm: Usually regular, but may be irregular.

Pacemaker Site: An ectopic pacemaker in the atria.

F Waves: Identical sawtooth-shaped repetitive waves.

FR Intervals: Usually equal, but may be unequal.

R-R Intervals: Usually equal and constant, but may be unequal.

QRS Complexes: Usually normal (0.10 sec or less), unless a preexisting intraventricular conduction disturbance, aberrant ventricular conduction, or ventricular preexcitation is present.

Treatment: See Section II, pages 45 and 49.

ATRIAL FIBRILLATION (AF)

Heart Rate: *Atrial rate:* 350-600 or more (average, 400) f waves/min. *Ventricular rate:* Usually 160-180/min if atrial fibrillation is uncontrolled (untreated); 60-70/min if controlled (treated) or if a preexisting AV block is present.

Rhythm: Irregularly (grossly) irregular.

Pacemaker Site: Multiple ectopic pacemakers in the atria.

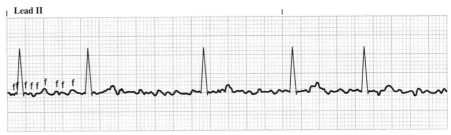

f Waves: Irregularly shaped, rounded (or pointed), and dissimilar atrial fibrillation (f) waves. If the f waves are large (≥1 mm), "coarse" fibrillatory waves are present; if they are small (<1 mm), "fine" fibrillatory waves are present.

fR Intervals: None.

R-R Intervals: Typically unequal.

QRS Complexes: Usually normal (0.10 sec or less), unless a preexisting intraventricular conduction disturbance, aberrant ventricular conduction, or ventricular preexcitation is present.

Treatment: See Section II, pages 45, 48, 49, and 50.

JUNCTIONAL ESCAPE RHYTHM

Heart Rate: 40-60/min, but may be less.

Rhythm: Essentially regular.

Pacemaker Site: An escape pacemaker in the AV junction.

P' Waves: P waves may be present or absent. If present, they either (1) regularly precede or follow each QRS complex, in which case, they are negative (inverted) in lead II having originated in the AV junction (P' waves), or

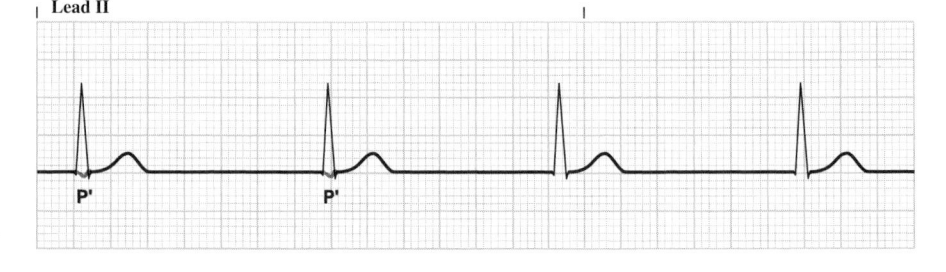

(2) occur independently, being either positive (upright) or negative (inverted) in lead II. If the P waves occur independently of the QRS complexes, AV dissociation is present. The pacemaker site of such P waves is the SA node or an ectopic pacemaker in the atria.

P'R/RP' Intervals: If the P' waves regularly precede the QRS complexes, the P'R intervals are abnormal (less than 0.12 sec). If the P' waves regularly follow the QRS complexes, the RP' intervals are less than 0.20 second.

R-R Intervals: Usually equal.

QRS Complexes: Usually normal (0.10 sec or less), unless a preexisting intraventricular conduction disturbance is present.

Treatment: See Section II, page 38.

PREMATURE JUNCTIONAL CONTRACTIONS (PJCs)

Heart Rate: That of the underlying rhythm.

Rhythm: Irregular when PJCs are present.

Pacemaker Site: An ectopic pacemaker in the AV junction.

P' Waves: P' waves may or may not be associated with the PJCs. If present, they usually differ from the P waves of the underlying rhythm in size, shape, and direction. The P' waves are nega-

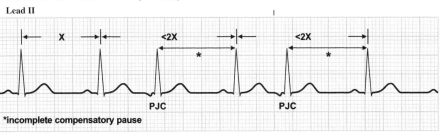

*incomplete compensatory pause

tive (inverted) in lead II. They may precede, be buried in, or, less commonly, follow the QRS complexes of the PJCs. P' waves followed or preceded by QRS complexes related to them are *conducted PJCs;* those occurring alone, not followed or preceded by QRS complexes, are *nonconducted* or *blocked PJCs.*

P'R/RP' Intervals: If P' waves regularly precede the QRS complexes of the PJCs, the P'R intervals are abnormal (less than 0.12 sec).

If P' waves regularly follow the QRS complexes, the RP' intervals are less than 0.20 second.

R-R Intervals: Unequal when PJCs are present. The pre-PJC R-R interval is shorter and the post-PJC R-R interval is longer than the R-R interval of the underlying rhythm. Commonly, a complete compensatory pause is present (i.e., the sum of the pre- and post-PJC R-R intervals is twice the R-R interval of the underlying rhythm). When the sum is less than twice the R-R interval of the underlying rhythm (uncommonly), an incomplete compensatory (or noncompensatory) pause is present.

QRS Complexes: The QRS complexes of the PJCs occur earlier than the next expected QRS complex of the underlying rhythm. Usually they are normal (0.10 sec or less), resembling those of the underlying rhythm. If aberrant ventricular conduction is present, the PJC may be wide and bizarre, resembling a PVC—PJC with aberrancy.

Treatment: See Section II, page 57.

TYPES OF PJCs

Infrequent PJCs: Less than five PJCs/min.

Frequent PJCs: Five or more PJCs/min.

Isolated PJCs (Beats): PJCs occurring singly.

Group Beats: PJCs occurring in groups of two or more.

Paired PJCs (Couplet): Two PJCs in a row.

Junctional Tachycardia: Three or more PJCs in a row.

Junctional Bigeminy: PJCs alternating with the QRS complexes of the underlying rhythm.

Junctional Trigeminy/Quadrigeminy: PJCs following every two or three QRS complexes of the underlying rhythm, respectively.

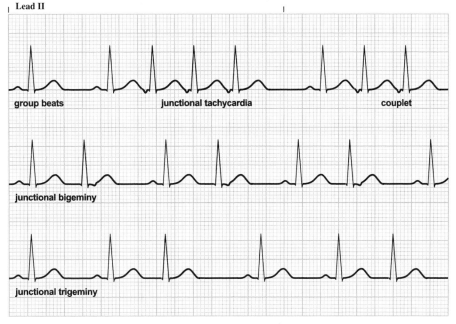

Lead II

group beats   junctional tachycardia   couplet

junctional bigeminy

junctional trigeminy

— = PJCs

NONPAROXYSMAL JUNCTIONAL TACHYCARDIA
(ACCELERATED JUNCTIONAL RHYTHM, JUNCTIONAL TACHYCARDIA)

Heart Rate: Usually 60-130/min, but may be as high as 150/min. Accelerated junctional rhythm: 60-100/min. Junctional tachycardia: 100/min or greater. Onset and termination are usually gradual.

Rhythm: Essentially regular.

Pacemaker Site: An ectopic pacemaker in the AV junction.

P Waves: P waves may be present or absent. If present, they either (1) regularly precede or follow each QRS complex, in which case they are negative (inverted) in lead II, having originated in the AV junction (P′ waves), or (2) occur independently, being either positive (upright) or negative (inverted) in lead II. If the P waves occur independently of the QRS complexes, AV dissociation is present. The pacemaker site of such P waves is the SA node or an ectopic pacemaker in the atria.

P′R/RP′ Intervals: If P′ waves regularly precede the QRS complexes, the P′R intervals are abnormal (less than 0.12 sec). If P′ waves

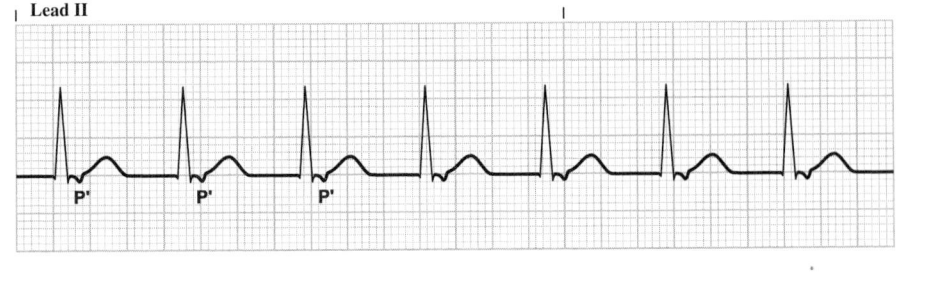

| Lead II

regularly follow the QRS complexes, the RP′ intervals are less than 0.20 second.

R-R Intervals: Usually equal.

QRS Complexes: Usually normal (0.10 sec or less), unless a preexisting intraventricular conduction disturbance or an aberrant ventricular conduction is present.

Treatment: No specific treatment indicated.

PAROXYSMAL SUPRAVENTRICULAR TACHYCARDIA (PSVT)

Heart Rate: Usually 160-240/min. PSVT occurs in paroxysms, beginning abruptly and lasting a few seconds to many hours.

Rhythm: Essentially regular.

Pacemaker Site: A reentry mechanism in the AV junction involving the AV node alone (AV nodal reentry tachycardia [AVNRT]) or the AV node and an accessory conduction pathway (AV reentry tachycardia [AVRT]).

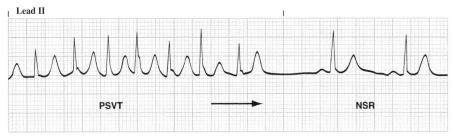

P′ Waves: Present or absent. When present, the P′ waves usually follow the QRS complexes; rarely they precede the QRS complexes. The P′ waves are generally negative (inverted) in lead II.

P′R/RP′ Intervals: If the P′ waves precede each QRS complex, the P′R intervals are abnormal (less than 0.12 sec). If the P′ waves follow each QRS complex, the RP′ intervals are less than 0.20 second. The P′R and RP′ intervals are usually constant.

R-R Intervals: Usually equal.

QRS Complexes: Usually normal (0.10 sec or less), unless a preexisting intraventricular conduction disturbance or an aberrant ventricular conduction is present. If the wide and bizarre QRS complexes occur only with the PSVT, the arrhythmia is called *PSVT with aberrancy* (or *PSVT with aberrant ventricular conduction*). Such a PSVT may resemble ventricular tachycardia.

Treatment: See Section II, page 42.

VENTRICULAR ESCAPE RHYTHM

Heart Rate: Usually 30-40/min, but may be less.

Rhythm: Regular, but may be irregular.

Pacemaker Site: An escape pacemaker in the ventricles.

P Waves: P waves may be present or absent. If present, they usually bear no relation to the QRS complexes, marching between and through them. Such P waves originate in the SA node or an ectopic pacemaker in the atria or AV junction. Uncommonly, negative P′ waves related to the arrythmia regularly follow the QRS complexes.

RP′ Intervals: Present if the P′ waves are associated with the PVCs, typically following them; about 0.20 second.

R-R Intervals: Usually equal, but may, be slightly unequal.

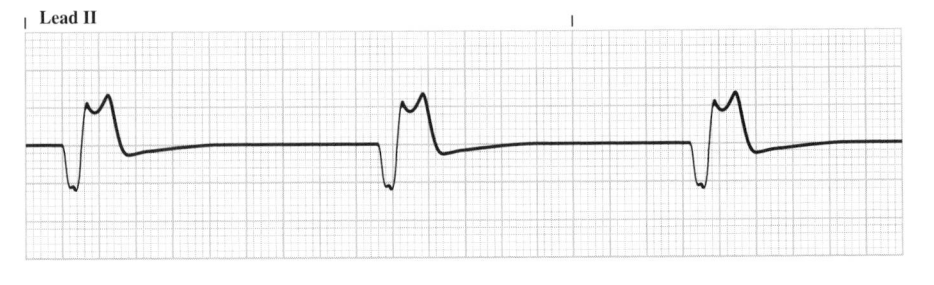

Lead II

QRS Complexes: Typically, wide (0.12 sec or greater) and bizarre. Usually identical, but may vary slightly.

Treatment: See Section II, page 38.

ACCELERATED IDIOVENTRICULAR RHYTHM (AIVR)

Heart Rate: 40-100/min.

Rhythm: Regular, but may be irregular.

Pacemaker Site: An ectopic pacemaker in the ventricles.

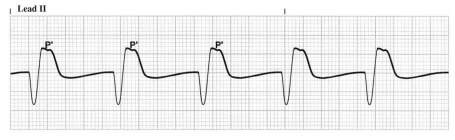

Lead II

P Waves: P waves may be present or absent. If present, they usually bear no relation to the QRS complexes, occurring independently of the QRS complexes. Such P waves originate in the SA node or an ectopic pacemaker in the atria or AV junction. Uncommonly, negative P' waves related to the arrhythmia regularly follow the QRS complexes.

RP' Intervals: Present if the P' waves are associated with the PVCs, typically following them; about 0.20 second.

R-R Intervals: Usually equal, but may be slightly unequal.

QRS Complexes: Typically wide (0.12 sec or greater) and bizarre. Usually identical, but may vary slightly.

Treatment: Usually no specific treatment indicated.

PREMATURE VENTRICULAR CONTRACTIONS (PVCs)

Heart Rate: That of the underlying rhythm.

Rhythm: Irregular when PVCs are present.

Pacemaker Site: An ectopic pacemaker in the ventricles.

P Waves: P waves may be present or absent. If present, they are usually of the underlying rhythm and bear no relation to the PVCs, sometimes appearing as notches in the ST segment or T wave of the PVCs. Uncommonly, the P' waves are related to the PVCs, in which case they follow the QRS complexes of the PVCs, appearing as negative (inverted) P' waves or notches in the ST segments or T waves of the PVCs in lead II.

RP' Intervals: Present if the P' waves are associated with the PVCs, typically following them; about 0.20 second.

R-R Intervals: Unequal when PVCs are present. The coupling interval, the interval between the PVC and the preceding QRS complex of the underlying rhythm, is shorter and the post-PVC R-R interval is longer than the R-R interval of the underlying rhythm. Commonly, a complete compensatory pause is present (i.e., the sum of the coupling interval and the post-PVC R-R interval is twice the R-R interval of the underlying rhythm). Rarely, when the sum is less than twice the R-R interval of the underlying rhythm, an incomplete compensatory pause is present.

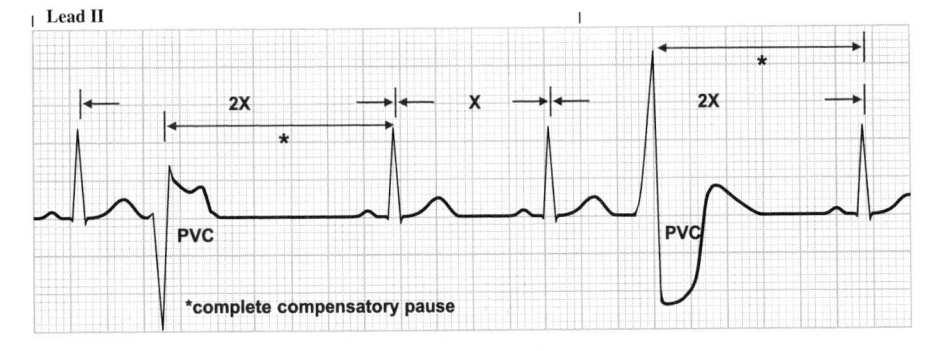

QRS Complexes: Typically wide (0.12 sec or greater) and bizarre. Identical PVCs are called *uniform PVCs*. PVCs with different QRS complexes are called *multiform PVCs*. PVCs with the same coupling intervals, indicating a single pacemaker site, are called *unifocal PVCs;* those with varying coupling intervals, indicating two or more pace-maker sites, are *multifocal PVCs*. Usually, uniform PVCs are unifocal, whereas multiform PVCs are multifocal but can be unifocal.

Treatment: See Section II, page 57.

TYPES OF PVCs

Infrequent PVCs: Less than five PVCs/min.

Frequent PVCs: Five or more PVCs/min.

Isolated PVCs (Beats): PVCs occurring singly.

Group Beats, Bursts, Salvos: PVCs occurring in groups of two or more.

Paired PVCs (Couplet): Two PVCs in a row.

Ventricular Tachycardia: Three or more PVCs in a row.

Ventricular Bigeminy: PVCs alternating with the QRS complexes of the underlying rhythm.

Ventricular Trigeminy/Ventricular Quadrigeminy: PVCs following every two or three QRS complexes of the underlying rhythm, respectively.

R-on-T Phenomenon: A PVC occurring during the downslope of the preceding T wave (vulnerable period of ventricular repolarization).

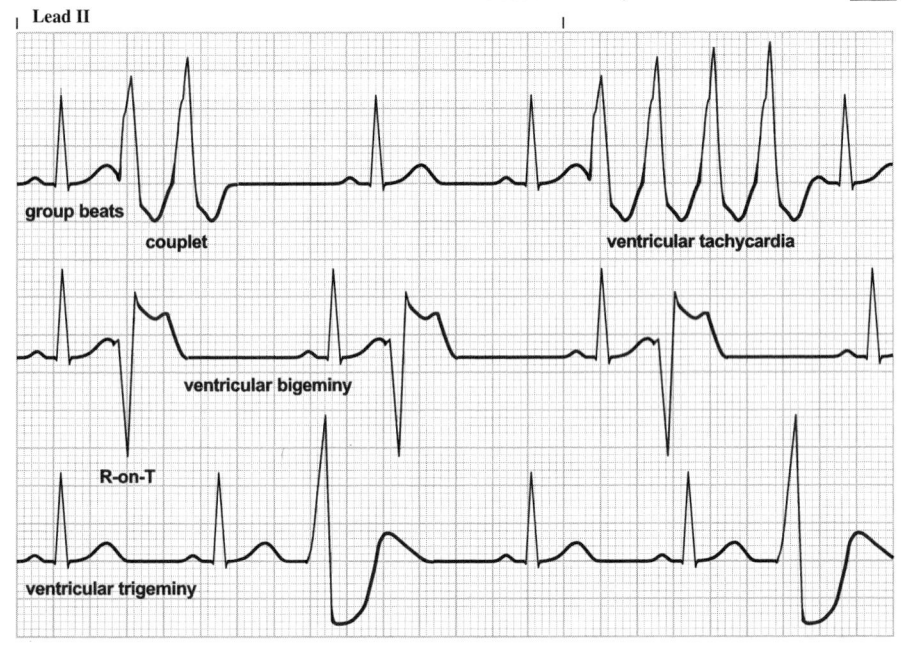

— = PVCs

VENTRICULAR TACHYCARDIA (VT)

Heart Rate: Usually 110-250/min.

Rhythm: Usually regular, but may be slightly irregular.

Pacemaker Site: An ectopic pacemaker in the ventricles.

P Waves: P waves may be present or absent. If present, they usually bear no relation to the QRS complexes, sometimes appearing here and there as notches in and between the ventricular complexes of the VT. Such P waves originate in the SA node or an ectopic pacemaker in the atria or AV junction. Uncommonly, the P′ waves are related to the VT, in which case they regularly appear as negative (inverted) P′ waves or notches in the latter part of the ventricular complexes or in between them, in lead II.

RP′ Intervals: Present if P′ waves regularly follow the QRS complexes; about 0.20 second.

R-R Intervals: Usually equal, but may be slightly unequal.

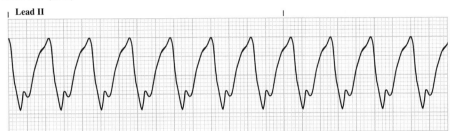

Lead II

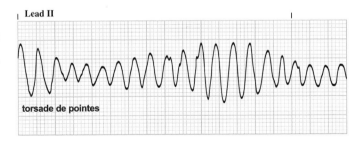

Lead II

torsade de pointes

QRS Complexes: Typically wide (0.12 sec or greater) and bizarre. Usually identical, but may vary slightly *(monomorphic VT)*. Two distinctly different QRS complexes alternating with each other indicate a *bidirectional VT*. When the QRS complexes vary greatly, *polymorphic VT* is present. When the QRS complexes gradually change back and forth from one shape and direction to another over a series of beats, the VT is called *torsade de pointes*.

Treatment: See Section II, pages 52, 54, 56, and 58.

VENTRICULAR FIBRILLATION (VF)

Heart Rate: 300-500/min.

Rhythm: Grossly (totally) irregular.

Pacemaker Site: Multiple ectopic pacemakers in the ventricles.

P Waves: None.

PR Intervals: None.

R-R Intervals: None.

QRS Complexes: Irregularly shaped, rounded (or pointed), and markedly dissimilar fibrillation (f) waves. If the f waves are large (>3 mm), "coarse" ventricular fibrillation is present; if the f waves are small (<3 mm), "fine" ventricular fibrillation is present.

Treatment: See Section II, page 58.

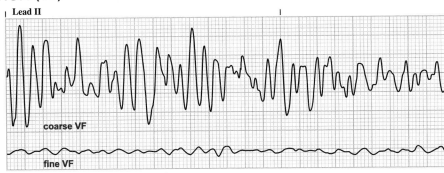

Lead II

coarse VF

fine VF

defib
v. fib

VENTRICULAR ASYSTOLE

Heart Rate: None.

Rhythm: None.

Pacemaker Site: None.

P Waves: P waves may be present or absent.

PR Intervals: None.

R-R Intervals: None.

QRS Complexes: None.

Treatment: See Section II, page 59.

Lead II

FIRST-DEGREE AV BLOCK

Heart Rate: The atrial and ventricular rates are typically the same.

Rhythm: That of the underlying rhythm.

P Waves: Those of the underlying rhythm; usually a QRS complex follows each P wave.

PR Intervals: Abnormal (greater than 0.20 sec); usually do not vary from beat to beat.

R-R Intervals: Those of the underlying rhythm.

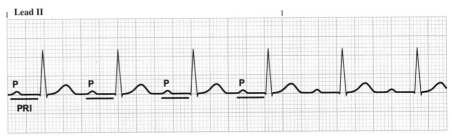

Lead II

QRS Complexes: Usually normal (0.10 sec or less), unless a preexisting intraventricular conduction disturbance is present.

AV Conduction Ratio: The AV conduction ratio is 1:1.

Treatment: No specific treatment indicated.

SECOND-DEGREE AV BLOCK
TYPE I AV BLOCK (WENCKEBACH)

Heart Rate: The atrial rate is that of the underlying rhythm. The ventricular rate is typically less than the atrial rate.

Rhythm: The atrial rhythm is essentially regular; the ventricular rhythm is usually irregular.

P Waves: Those of the underlying rhythm; periodically a QRS complex fails to occur after a P wave (nonconducted P wave or dropped beat).

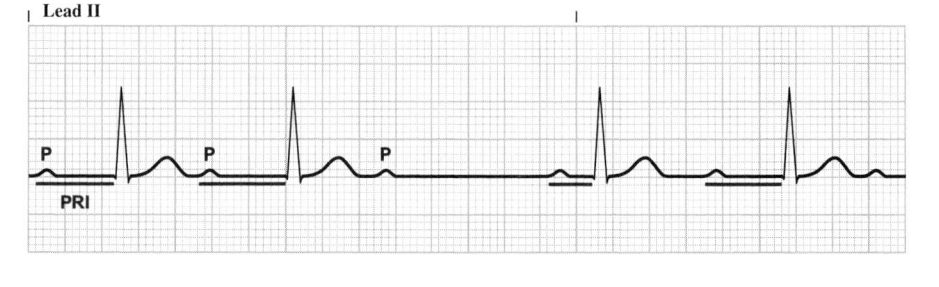

PR Intervals: Gradually lengthen until a dropped beat occurs, after which the sequence begins anew.

R-R Intervals: Unequal; gradually decrease as the PR intervals lengthen until a dropped beat occurs, resulting in a prolonged R-R interval. Following this, the cycle begins anew.

QRS Complexes: Usually normal (0.10 sec or less), unless a preexisting intraventricular conduction disturbance is present.

AV Conduction Ratio: Commonly, the AV conduction ratio is 5:4, 4:3, or 3:2, but it may be 6:5, 7:6, and so forth.

Treatment: See Section II, page 36.

SECOND-DEGREE AV BLOCK, TYPE II AV BLOCK

Heart Rate: The atrial rate is that of the underlying rhythm. The ventricular rate is typically less than the atrial rate.

Rhythm: The atrial rhythm is essentially regular; the ventricular rhythm is usually irregular.

P Waves: Those of the underlying rhythm; periodically a QRS complex fails to occur after a P wave (nonconducted P wave or dropped beat).

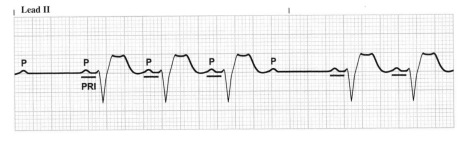

PR Intervals: May be normal (0.12-0.20 sec) or abnormal (greater than 0.20 sec); usually constant.

R-R Intervals: Unequal.

QRS Complexes: Typically, abnormal (greater than 0.12 sec) because of a bundle branch block; rarely, normal (0.10 sec or less).

AV Conduction Ratio: The AV conduction ratio is commonly 4:3 or 3:2, but it may be 5:4, 6:5, 7:6, and so forth.

Treatment: See Section II, page 37.

SECOND-DEGREE AV BLOCK
2:1 AND ADVANCED AV BLOCK

Heart Rate: The atrial rate is that of the underlying rhythm. The ventricular rate is typically less than the atrial rate.

Rhythm: The atrial rhythm is essentially regular; the ventricular rhythm may be regular or irregular.

P Waves: Those of the underlying rhythm; periodically, QRS complexes fail to occur after one or more P waves (nonconducted P waves or dropped beats).

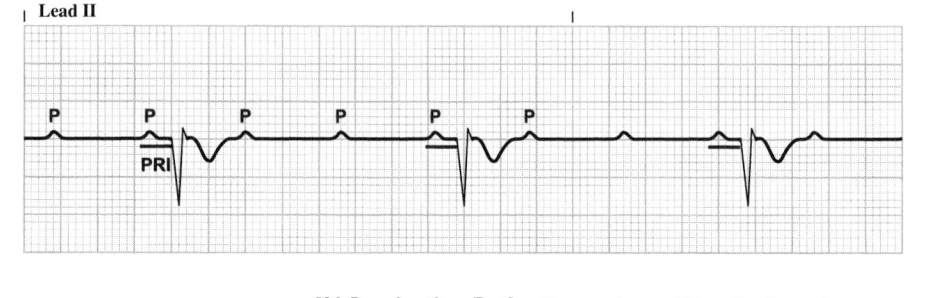

Lead II

PR Intervals: Normal (0.12-0.20 sec) or abnormal (greater than 0.20 sec); usually constant.

R-R Intervals: Equal or may vary.

QRS Complexes: Normal (0.10 sec or less) or abnormal (greater than 0.12 sec) because of a bundle branch block.

AV Conduction Ratio: Commonly, the AV conduction ratios are even numbers, 2:1, 4:1, 6:1, 8:1, and so forth, but they may be uneven numbers, 3:1 or 5:1. A 3:1 or higher AV block is called an *advanced AV block.*

Treatment: See Section II, page 36.

THIRD-DEGREE AV BLOCK

Heart Rate: The atrial rate is that of the underlying rhythm. The ventricular rate is typically 40-60/min (but may be 30-40/min or less) and independent of the atrial rate (i.e., AV dissociation).

Rhythm: The atrial rhythm is that of the underlying rhythm: regular or irregular. The ventricular rhythm is essentially regular.

Pacemaker Site: The pacemaker site of the P waves is the SA node or an ectopic pacemaker in the atria or AV junction. The pacemaker site of the QRS complexes is an escape pacemaker in the AV junction (junctional escape rhythm) or ventricles (ventricular escape rhythm).

P Waves: The P waves occur independently of the QRS complexes.

PR Intervals: None.

R-R Intervals: Usually equal.

QRS Complexes: May be normal (0.10 sec or less) or abnormal (greater than 0.12 sec).

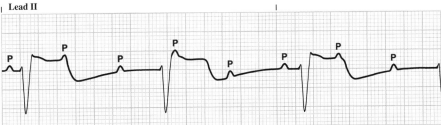

Lead II

Treatment: See Section II, pages 36 and 37.

Arrhythmia Management

SINUS BRADYCARDIA
SINUS ARREST/SINOATRIAL (SA) EXIT BLOCK
SECOND-DEGREE, TYPE I AV BLOCK (WENCKEBACH)
SECOND-DEGREE, 2:1 AND ADVANCED AV BLOCK WITH NARROW QRS COMPLEXES
THIRD-DEGREE AV BLOCK WITH NARROW QRS COMPLEXES

A. Asymptomatic
◆ No specific treatment indicated.

B. Symptomatic*
◆ Administer an **atropine** 0.5 IV/IO bolus rapidly. Repeat every 3 to 5 min until the heart rate is 60 to 100/min or the maximum dose of 3 mg (0.04 mg/kg) of atropine has been administered.

AND/OR

Initiate transcutaneous pacing. If the patient has discomfort and is not hypotensive, administer a sedative such as **midazolam** or **diazepam** as follows:

◆ Midazolam 1 to 2 mg IV slowly over at least 2 min and repeat every 3 to 5 min, titrated to produce sedation/amnesia

OR

Diazepam 5 to 15 mg with or without 2 to 5 mg **morphine** IV slowly to produce amnesia/analgesia
◆ Prepare for immediate transvenous pacing.

If symptomatic bradycardia and/or hypotension persist, increase the heart rate to 60 to 100/min and the systolic blood pressure to within normal limits by administering:

◆ **Dopamine hydrochloride** IV infusion at a rate of 5 to 20 μg/kg/min

OR

　Epinephrine IV infusion at a rate of 2 to 10 μg/min

---

*A bradycardia is considered "symptomatic" when one or more of the following clinical conditions or signs or symptoms are present:
◆ Hypotension or shock (systolic blood pressure less than 90 mm Hg)
◆ Congestive heart failure, pulmonary congestion
◆ Chest pain or dyspnea
◆ Decreased level of consciousness caused by decreased cardiac output
◆ PVCs, particularly in the setting of an acute myocardial infarction (MI)

SECOND-DEGREE, TYPE II AV BLOCK
SECOND-DEGREE, 2:1 AND ADVANCED AV BLOCK WITH WIDE QRS COMPLEXES
THIRD-DEGREE AV BLOCK WITH WIDE QRS COMPLEXES

A. Asymptomatic, in the presence of acute anterior MI involving the interventricular septum

- Attach a transcutaneous pacemaker, and put on standby.

B. Symptomatic

- Initiate transcutaneous pacing. If the patient has discomfort and is not hypotensive, administer a sedative such as **midazolam** or **diazepam** as follows:
  - ◇ Midazolam 1 to 2 mg IV slowly over at least 2 min and repeat every 3 to 5 min, titrated to produce sedation/amnesia

    OR

    Diazepam 5 to 15 mg with or without 2 to 5 mg **morphine** IV slowly to produce amnesia/analgesia

- Prepare for immediate transvenous pacing.

If symptomatic bradycardia and/or hypotension persist, increase the heart rate to 60 to 100/min and the systolic blood pressure to within normal limits by administering:

- **Dopamine hydrochloride** IV infusion at a rate of 5 to 20 μg/kg/min

    OR

    Epinephrine IV infusion at a rate of 2 to 10 μg/min

JUNCTIONAL ESCAPE RHYTHM
VENTRICULAR ESCAPE RHYTHM

A. Asymptomatic
- No specific treatment indicated.

B. Symptomatic
- Initiate transcutaneous pacing. If the patient has discomfort and is not hypotensive, administer a sedative such as **midazolam** or **diazepam** as follows:
  - ◇ Midazolam 1 to 2 mg IV slowly over at least 2 min and repeat every 3 to 5 min, titrated to produce sedation/amnesia

    OR

    Diazepam 5 to 15 mg with or without 2 to 5 mg **morphine** IV slowly to produce amnesia/analgesia
  - ◇ Consider atropine 0.5 mg IV/IO.
    May repeat to a total dose of 3.0 mg IV/IO.
- Prepare for immediate transvenous pacing.

If symptomatic bradycardia and/or hypotension persist, increase the heart rate to 60 to 100/min and the systolic blood pressure to within normal limits by administering:
- **Dopamine hydrochloride** IV infusion at a rate of 5 to 20 μg/kg/min

  OR

  Epinephrine IV infusion at a rate of 2 to 10 μg/min

SINUS TACHYCARDIA

A. Patient's condition stable or unstable*
- No specific treatment indicated.
- Treat underlying cause:
  - ◇ Anxiety, exercise, pain, fever
  - ◇ Congestive heart failure, hypoxemia
  - ◇ Hypovolemia, hypotension, shock
- Discontinue such drugs as:
  - ◇ Atropine
  - ◇ Epinephrine, vasopressors

---

*A patient's condition is considered "unstable" when one or more of the following clinical conditions or signs or symptoms are present:
- Hypotension or shock (systolic blood pressure 90 mm Hg or less)
- Congestive heart failure, pulmonary congestion
- Chest pain or dyspnea
- Decreased level of consciousness caused by decreased cardiac output
- Acute MI

ATRIAL TACHYCARDIA WITH BLOCK

A. Patient's condition stable or unstable

- No specific treatment indicated.
- Treat underlying cause.
- Discontinue digitalis, if digitalis toxicity is suspected.

NARROW-QRS-COMPLEX TACHYCARDIA OF UNKNOWN ORIGIN (WITH PULSE)

A. Patient's condition stable

- Perform vagal maneuvers.
- Administer an **adenosine** 6-mg IV bolus rapidly, followed by a 20-mL flush of IV fluid, and in 1 to 2 min, if necessary, repeat adenosine 12 mg rapidly, followed by an IV flush. Repeat once in 1 to 2 min, if necessary.
- Determine if arrhythmia is:
  - Atrial tachycardia without block
  - Paroxysmal supraventricular tachycardia (PSVT)
  - Junctional tachycardia

ATRIAL TACHYCARDIA WITHOUT BLOCK

A. Patient's condition stable and heart rate over 150 beats/min

- Establish IV/IO access.
- Obtain 12-lead ECG.
- Attempt vagal maneuvers.
- Adenosine 6 mg IV/IO push. Repeat at 12 mg IV/IO push; may repeat once.
- Administer a **calcium channel blocker if not contraindicated.**
  - ◇ **Diltiazem** 20 mg (0.25 mg/kg) IV slowly over 2 min. In 15 min, if necessary and no adverse effects, repeat diltiazem 25 mg (0.35 mg/kg). Follow by an IV infusion at a rate of 5 to 15 mg/h.

  OR
- Administer one of the following β-blockers:
  - ◇ **Esmolol** 0.5-mg/kg IV bolus over 1 min, followed by an IV infusion at a rate of 0.05 mg/kg/min and repeat the IV bolus twice, 5 min between each bolus, while increasing the rate of the IV infusion 0.05 mg/kg/min after each bolus. Then, if necessary, increase the IV infusion by 0.05 mg/kg/min every 5 min to a maximum of 0.30 mg/kg/min.
  - ◇ **Atenolol** 5 mg IV over 5 min and repeat in 10 min for a total dose of 10 mg

  - ◇ **Metoprolol** 5 mg IV over 2 to 5 min and repeat every 5 min up to a total dose of 15 mg

  OR
- Administer an antiarrhythmic drug such as **amiodarone.**
  - ◇ Amiodarone 150-mg IV infusion over 10 min, followed by a 1-mg/min IV infusion

B. Patient's condition unstable and heart rate over 150 beats/min or less

- Perform immediate synchronized cardioversion.
- Establish IV access, sedate if patient is conscious.
- Do not delay cardioversion.
- Administer an antiarrhythmic drug such as **amiodarone.**
  - ◇ Amiodarone 150-mg IV infusion over 10 min, followed by a 1-mg/min IV infusion

  OR
- Administer a **calcium channel blocker.**
  - ◇ **Diltiazem** 20 mg (0.25 mg/kg) IV slowly over 2 min. In 15 min, if necessary and no adverse effects, repeat diltiazem 25 mg (0.35 mg/kg). Follow by an IV infusion at a rate of 5 to 15 mg/h.

Caution!

Calcium channel blockers are contraindicated:

♦ If hypotension or cardiogenic shock is present
♦ If second- or third-degree AV block, sinus node dysfunction, atrial flutter or fibrillation associated with Wolff-Parkinson-White conduction, or a wide-QRS-complex tachycardia is present
♦ If β-blockers are being administered intravenously, or
♦ If there is a history of bradycardia.

Calcium channel blockers should be used cautiously, if at all, in congestive heart failure and in patients receiving oral β-blockers.

The patient's blood pressure and pulse must be monitored frequently during and after the administration of a calcium channel blocker.

If hypotension occurs with a calcium channel blocker, place the patient in a Trendelenburg position and administer 1 g of calcium chloride IV slowly, IV fluids, and a vasopressor.

If bradycardia, AV block, or asystole occurs, refer to the appropriate treatment protocol.

Caution!

β-blockers are contraindicated:

♦ If bradycardia (heart rate <60 bpm) is present
♦ If hypotension (systolic blood pressure <100 mm Hg) is present
♦ If PR interval >0.24 second or second- or third-degree AV block is present
♦ If congestive heart failure (left and/or right heart failure) is present
♦ If bronchospasm or a history of asthma is present
♦ If severe chronic obstructive pulmonary disease (COPD) is present, or
♦ If intravenous calcium channel blockers have been administered within a few hours

The patient's blood pressure and pulse must be monitored frequently during and after the administration of a β-blocker.

If hypotension occurs with a β-blocker, place the patient in a Trendelenburg position and administer a vasopressor.

If bradycardia, AV block, or asystole occurs, refer to the appropriate treatment protocol.

PAROXYSMAL SUPRAVENTRICULAR TACHYCARDIA (PSVT) WITH NARROW QRS COMPLEXES
(WITHOUT WOLFF-PARKINSON-WHITE SYNDROME OR VENTRICULAR PREEXCITATION)

A. Patient's condition stable and heart rate over 150 beats/min

- Perform vagal maneuvers.
- Administer an **adenosine** 6-mg IV bolus rapidly, followed by a 20-mL flush of IV fluid, and in 1 to 2 min, if necessary, repeat adenosine 12 mg rapidly, followed by an IV flush. Repeat once in 1 to 2 min, if necessary.
- Administer a **calcium channel blocker.**
  - ⬦ **Diltiazem** 20 mg (0.25 mg/kg) IV slowly over 2 min. In 15 min, if necessary and no adverse effects, repeat diltiazem 25 mg (0.35 mg/kg). Follow by an IV infusion at a rate of 5 to 15 mg/h.

    OR
- Administer one of the following **β-blockers:**
  - ⬦ **Esmolol** 0.5-mg/kg IV bolus over 1 min, followed by an IV infusion at a rate of 0.05 mg/kg/min and repeat the IV bolus twice, 5 min between each bolus, while increasing the rate of the IV infusion 0.05 mg/kg/min after each bolus. Then, if necessary, increase the IV infusion by 0.05 mg/kg/min every 5 min to a maximum of 0.30 mg/kg/min.
  - ⬦ **Atenolol** 5 mg IV over 5 min and repeat in 10 min for a total dose of 10 mg
  - ⬦ **Metoprolol** 5 mg IV over 2 to 5 min and repeat every 5 min up to a total dose of 15 mg
- Administer an initial dose of **digoxin** 0.5 mg IV over 5 min.
- Establish IV access, sedate if patient is conscious.
- Cardiovert at 50-100 J with a monophasic waveform.
- Escalate subsequent shock doses as required.

B. Patient's condition unstable and heart rate over 150 beats/min or less

◆ Establish IV access, sedate if patient is conscious.
◆ Cardiovert at 50-100 J with a monophasic waveform.
◆ Escalate subsequent shock doses as required.
◆ Administer an antiarrhythmic drug such as **amiodarone.**
  ◇ Amiodarone 150-mg IV infusion over 10 min, followed by a 1-mg/min IV infusion

OR

◆ Administer a **calcium channel blocker.**
  ◇ **Diltiazem** 20 mg (0.25 mg/kg) IV slowly over 2 min. In 15 min, if necessary and no adverse effects, repeat diltiazem 25 mg (0.35 mg/kg). Follow by an IV infusion at a rate of 5 to 15 mg/h.

JUNCTIONAL TACHYCARDIA

A. Patient's condition stable and heart rate over 150 beats/min

- Administer an antiarrhythmic drug such as **amiodarone.**
  - ◇ Amiodarone 150-mg IV infusion over 10 min, followed by a 1-mg/min IV infusion

OR

- Administer one of the following β-blockers:
  - ◇ **Esmolol** 0.5-mg/kg IV bolus over 1 min, followed by an IV infusion at a rate of 0.05 mg/kg/min and repeat the IV bolus twice, 5 min between each bolus, while increasing the rate of the IV infusion 0.05 mg/kg/min after each bolus. Then, if necessary, increase the IV infusion by 0.05 mg/kg/min every 5 min to a maximum of 0.30 mg/kg/min.
  - ◇ **Atenolol** 5 mg IV over 5 min and repeat in 10 min for a total dose of 10 mg
  - ◇ **Metoprolol** 5 mg IV over 2 to 5 min and repeat every 5 min up to a total dose of 15 mg

B. Patient's condition unstable and heart rate over 150 beats/min or less

- Establish IV access, sedate if patient is conscious.
- Cardiovert at 50-100 J with a monophasic waveform.
- Escalate subsequent shock doses as required.
- Administer an antiarrhythmic drug such as **amiodarone.**
  - ◇ Amiodarone 150-mg IV infusion over 10 min, followed by a 1-mg/min IV infusion

ATRIAL FLUTTER/ATRIAL FIBRILLATION
(WITHOUT WOLFF-PARKINSON-WHITE SYNDROME OR VENTRICULAR PREEXCITATION)

Treatment to Control the Heart Rate

A. Patient's condition stable and heart rate over 120 beats/min

- Administer one of the following β-blockers:
  - **Esmolol** 0.5-mg/kg IV bolus over 1 min, followed by an IV infusion at a rate of 0.05 mg/kg/min and repeat the IV bolus twice, 5 min between each bolus, while increasing the rate of the IV infusion 0.05 mg/kg/min after each bolus. Then, if necessary, increase the IV infusion by 0.05 mg/kg/min every 5 min to a maximum of 0.30 mg/kg/min.
  - **Atenolol** 5 mg IV over 5 min and repeat in 10 min for a total dose of 10 mg
  - **Metoprolol** 5 mg IV over 2 to 5 min and repeat every 5 min up to a total dose of 15 mg

OR

- Administer a **calcium channel blocker** if not contraindicated.
  - **Diltiazem** 20 mg (0.25 mg/kg) IV slowly over 2 min. In 15 min, if necessary and no adverse effects, repeat diltiazem 25 mg (0.35 mg/kg). Follow by an IV infusion at a rate of 5 to 15 mg/h.
- Administer an initial dose of **digoxin** 0.5 mg IV over 5 min.

B. Patient's condition unstable and heart rate over 120 beats/min or less

- Administer an initial dose of **digoxin** 0.5 mg IV over 5 min.
- Administer a **calcium channel blocker** if not contraindicated.
  - **Diltiazem** 20 mg (0.25 mg/kg) IV slowly over 2 min. In 15 min, if necessary and no adverse effects, repeat diltiazem 25 mg (0.35 mg/kg). Follow by an IV infusion at a rate of 5 to 15 mg/h.

OR

- Administer an antiarrhythmic drug such as **amiodarone,** but only if atrial fibrillation has been present for less than 48 hours.
  - **Amiodarone** 150-mg IV infusion over 10 min, followed by a 1-mg/min IV infusion

Treatment to Convert the Rhythm

Atrial Fibrillation <48 Hours and Atrial Flutter of Any Duration

A. Patient's condition stable and heart rate over 120 beats/min

- Administer a short-acting antiarrhythmic drug such as **ibutilide.**
  - If the patient weighs ≥60 kg (≥132 lb), administer 1 mg of ibutilide IV over 10 min and repeat in 10 min if necessary after completion of the first infusion.

⬥ If the patient weighs < 60 kg (<132 lb) administer 0.1 mg/kg of ibutilide IV over 10 min and repeat in 10 min if necessary after completion of the first infusion.

OR

Administer an antiarrhythmic drug such as **amiodarone.**
◆ Amiodarone 150-mg IV infusion over 10 min, followed by a 1-mg/min IV infusion

OR

If the antiarrhythmic drug is unsuccessful in converting atrial flutter or atrial fibrillation:
◆ Perform synchronized cardioversion

For Atrial Fib:	Cardiovert at 100 to 200 J with a monophasic waveform.
	Cardiovert at 100 to 120 J with a biphasic waveform.
	Escalate subsequent shock doses as required.
For Atrial Flutter:	Cardiovert at 50-100 J with a monophasic waveform.
	Escalate subsequent shock doses as required.

B. Patient's condition unstable and heart rate over 120 beats/min or less

Consider immediate DC cardioversion or administration of an antiarrhythmic drug.

- Perform synchronized cardioversion

For Atrial Fib:	Cardiovert at 100 to 200 J with a monophasic waveform.
	Cardiovert at 100 to 120 J with a biphasic waveform.
	Escalate subsequent shock doses as required.
For Atrial Flutter:	Cardiovert at 50 to 100 J with a monophasic waveform.
	Escalate subsequent shock doses as required.

- Administer an antiarrhythmic drug such as **amiodarone.**
  - ⋄ Amiodarone 150-mg IV infusion over 10 min, followed by a 1-mg/min IV infusion

If amiodarone is unsuccessful in converting atrial flutter or atrial fibrillation:

  - ⋄ Peform **DC cardioversion** as above.

ATRIAL FIBRILLATION
(WITHOUT WOLFF-PARKINSON-WHITE SYNDROME OR VENTRICULAR PREEXCITATION)

Treatment to Convert the Rhythm
Atrial Fibrillation >48 Hours or of Unknown Duration

A. Patient's condition stable and heart rate over 120 beats/min
- Administer one of the following β-blockers if not contraindicated:
  - **Esmolol** 0.5-mg/kg IV bolus over 1 min, followed by an IV infusion at a rate of 0.05 mg/kg/min and repeat the IV bolus twice, 5 min between each bolus, while increasing the rate of the IV infusion 0.05 mg/kg/min after each bolus. Then, if necessary, increase the IV infusion by 0.05 mg/kg/min every 5 min to a maximum of 0.30 mg/kg/min.
  - **Atenolol** 5 mg IV over 5 min and repeat in 10 min for a total dose of 10 mg
  - **Metoprolol** 5 mg IV over 2 to 5 min and repeat every 5 min up to a total dose of 15 mg

OR

- Administer a **calcium channel blocker** if not contraindicated.
  - **Diltiazem** 20 mg (0.25 mg/kg) IV slowly over 2 min. In 15 min, if necessary and no adverse effects, repeat diltiazem 25 mg (0.35 mg/kg). Follow by an IV infusion at a rate of 5 to 15 mg/h.
- Administer an initial dose of **digoxin** 0.5 mg IV over 5 min.
- Delay DC cardioversion until the patient is anticoagulated and atrial thrombi are excluded.

B. Patient's condition unstable and heart rate over 120 beats/min or less
- Administer a **calcium channel blocker** if not contraindicated.
  - **Diltiazem** 20 mg (0.25 mg/kg) IV slowly over 2 min. In 15 min, if necessary and no adverse effects, repeat diltiazem 25 mg (0.35 mg/kg). Follow by an IV infusion at a rate of 5 to 15 mg/h.
- Administer an initial dose of **digoxin** 0.5 mg IV over 5 min.
- Delay DC cardioversion until the patient is anticoagulated and atrial thrombi are excluded.

ATRIAL FLUTTER/ATRIAL FIBRILLATION (WITH WOLFF-PARKINSON-WHITE SYNDROME OR VENTRICULAR PREEXCITATION)

Treatment to Control the Heart Rate and/or Convert the Rhythm

Atrial Fibrillation <48 Hours and Atrial Flutter of Any Duration

A. Patient's condition stable and heart rate over 120 beats/min

- Administer an antiarrhythmic drug such as **amiodarone.**
  - Amiodarone 150-mg IV infusion over 10 min, followed by a 1-mg/min IV infusion

OR

- Administer an antiarrhythmic drug such as **procainamide hydrochloride** if not contraindicated.
  - Procainamide hydrochloride IV infusion at a rate of 20 to 30 mg/min until (1) the arrhythmia is suppressed, (2) a total dose of 17 mg/kg of procainamide has been administered, (3) side effects from procainamide appear, (4) the QRS complex widens by 50% of its original width, or (5) the PR or QT interval lengthens by 50% of its original length. If procainamide suppresses the arrhythmia, start a maintenance infusion of procainamide at a rate of 1 to 4 mg/min.

If one of the antiarrhythmic drugs is unsuccessful in converting atrial flutter or atrial fibrillation:

- Deliver a low-energy synchronized shock (50 or 100 J for atrial flutter, 100 or 200 J for atrial fibrillation) and repeat the synchronized shock as often as necessary at progressively increasing energy levels as appropriate (100 J, 200 J, and so forth, up to 360 J). In the conscious patient, premedicate the patient before cardioversion, using a sedative such as **midazolam** or **diazepam** as follows:
  - Midazolam 1 to 2 mg IV slowly over at least 2 min and repeat every 3 to 5 min, titrated to produce sedation/amnesia before cardioversion

OR

Diazepam 5 to 15 mg with or without 2 to 5 mg **morphine** IV slowly to produce amnesia/analgesia before cardioversion

B. Patient's condition unstable and heart rate over 120 beats/min or less

Consider immediate DC cardioversion or administration of an antiarrhythmic drug.

◆ Deliver a low-energy synchronized shock (50 or 100 J for atrial flutter, 100 or 200 J for atrial fibrillation) and repeat the synchronized shock as often as necessary at progressively increasing energy levels as appropriate (100 J, 200 J, and so forth, up to 360 J). In the conscious patient, premedicate the patient before cardioversion, using a sedative such as **midazolam** or **diazepam** as follows:

⬥ Midazolam 1 to 2 mg IV slowly over at least 2 min and repeat every 3 to 5 min, titrated to produce sedation/amnesia before cardioversion

OR

Diazepam 5 to 15 mg with or without 2 to 5 mg morphine IV slowly to produce amnesia/analgesia before cardioversion

◆ Administer an antiarrhythmic drug such as **amiodarone.**

⬥ Amiodarone 150-mg IV infusion over 10 min, followed by a 1-mg/min IV infusion

If amiodarone is unsuccessful in converting atrial flutter or atrial fibrillation:

⬥ Peform **DC cardioversion** as above.

ATRIAL FIBRILLATION
(WITH WOLFF-PARKINSON-WHITE SYNDROME OR VENTRICULAR PREEXCITATION)

Treatment to Control the Heart Rate and/or Convert the Rhythm

Atrial Fibrillation >48 Hours or of Unknown Duration

A. Patient's condition stable or unstable and heart rate over 120 beats/min or less (if unstable)

◆ Administer an antiarrhythmic drug such as **amiodarone** with caution.

⬥ Amiodarone 150-mg IV infusion over 10 min, followed by a 1-mg/min IV infusion

◆ Delay DC cardioversion until the patient is anticoagulated and atrial thrombi are excluded.

WIDE-QRS-COMPLEX TACHYCARDIA OF UNKNOWN ORIGIN (WITH PULSE)

A. Patient's condition stable

Consider immediate DC cardioversion or administration of an antiarrhythmic drug.

- Deliver a synchronized shock (100 J) (monophasic waveform) and repeat the synchronized shock as often as necessary at progressively increasing energy levels as appropriate (200 J, 300 J, and 360 J). In the conscious patient, premedicate the patient before cardioversion, using a sedative such as **midazolam** or **diazepam** as follows:
  - Midazolam 1 to 2 mg IV slowly over at least 2 min and repeat every 3 to 5 min, titrated to produce sedation/amnesia before cardioversion

  OR

  Diazepam 5 to 15 mg with or without 2 to 5 mg morphine IV slowly to produce amnesia/analgesia before cardioversion
- Administer an antiarrhythmic drug such as **amiodarone.**
  - Amiodarone 150-mg IV infusion over 10 min, followed by a 1-mg/min IV infusion

B. Patient's condition unstable

Consider immediate DC cardioversion or administration of an antiarrhythmic drug.

- Deliver a synchronized shock (100 J) (monophasic waveform) and repeat the synchronized shock as often as necessary at progressively increasing energy levels as appropriate (200 J, 300 J, and 360 J). In the conscious patient, premedicate the patient before cardioversion, using a sedative such as **midazolam** or **diazepam** as follows:
  - Midazolam 1 to 2 mg IV slowly over at least 2 min and repeat every 3 to 5 min, titrated to produce sedation/amnesia before cardioversion

  OR

  Diazepam 5 to 15 mg with or without 2 to 5 mg **morphine** IV slowly to produce amnesia/analgesia before cardioversion
- Administer an antiarrhythmic drug such as **amiodarone.**
  - Amiodarone 150-mg IV infusion over 10 min, followed by a 1-mg/min IV infusion

VENTRICULAR TACHYCARDIA (VT), MONOMORPHIC (WITH PULSE)

A. Patient's condition stable

Consider immediate DC cardioversion or administration of an antiarrhythmic drug.

- Administer an antiarrhythmic drug such as **amiodarone.**
  - ◇ Amiodarone 150-mg IV infusion over 10 min, followed by a 1-mg/min IV infusion

- Deliver a synchronized shock (100 J) and repeat the synchronized shock as often as necessary at progressively increasing energy levels as appropriate (200 J, 300 J, and 360 J). In the conscious patient, premedicate the patient before cardioversion, using a sedative such as **midazolam** or **diazepam** as follows:
  - ◇ Midazolam 1 to 2 mg IV slowly over at least 2 min and repeat every 3 to 5 min, titrated to produce sedation/amnesia before cardioversion

    OR

    Diazepam 5 to 15 mg with or without 2 to 5 mg **morphine** IV slowly to produce amnesia/analgesia before cardioversion

B. Patient's condition unstable

Consider immediate DC cardioversion or administration of an antiarrhythmic drug.

- ◆ Deliver a synchronized shock (100 J) and repeat the synchronized shock as often as necessary at progressively increasing energy levels as appropriate (200 J, 300 J, and 360 J). In the conscious patient, premedicate the patient before cardioversion, using a sedative such as **midazolam** or **diazepam** as follows:
  - ◇ Midazolam 1 to 2 mg IV slowly over at least 2 min and repeat every 3 to 5 min, titrated to produce sedation/amnesia before cardioversion

    OR

    Diazepam 5 to 15 mg with or without 2 to 5 mg **morphine** IV slowly to produce amnesia/analgesia before cardioversion

- ◆ Administer an antiarrhythmic drug such as **amiodarone.**
  - ◇ Amiodarone 150-mg IV infusion over 10 min, followed by a 1-mg/min IV infusion

VENTRICULAR TACHYCARDIA (VT), POLYMORPHIC (WITH PULSE) NORMAL BASELINE QT INTERVAL

A. Patient's condition stable

Consider immediate DC cardioversion or administration of an antiarrhythmic drug while correcting any electrolyte imbalance.

♦ Deliver a synchronized shock (100 J) and repeat the synchronized shock as often as necessary at progressively increasing energy levels as appropriate (200 J, 300 J, and 360 J). In the conscious patient, premedicate the patient before cardioversion, using a sedative such as **midazolam** or **diazepam** as follows:
  ◇ Midazolam 1 to 2 mg IV slowly over at least 2 min and repeat every 3 to 5 min, titrated to produce sedation/amnesia before cardioversion

  OR

  Diazepam 5 to 15 mg with or without 2 to 5 mg **morphine** IV slowly to produce amnesia/analgesia before cardioversion
♦ If the polymorphic VT is associated with an acute coronary syndrome, treat the acute coronary syndrome, while correcting the myocardial ischemia, as far as possible.

  AND

♦ Administer one of the following **β-blockers** if not contraindicated:
  ◇ **Esmolol** 0.5-mg/kg IV bolus over 1 min, followed by an IV infusion at a rate of 0.05 mg/kg/min and repeat the IV bolus twice, 5 min between each bolus, while increasing the rate of the IV infusion 0.05 mg/kg/min after each bolus. Then, if necessary, increase the IV infusion by 0.05 mg/kg/min every 5 min to a maximum of 0.30 mg/kg/min.
  ◇ **Atenolol** 5 mg IV over 5 min and repeat in 10 min for a total dose of 10 mg
  ◇ **Metoprolol** 5 mg IV over 2 to 5 min and repeat every 5 min up to a total dose of 15 mg

  OR

♦ If the polymorphic VT is or is not associated with an acute coronary syndrome, administer an antiarrhythmic drug such as **amiodarone.**
  ◇ Amiodarone 150-mg IV infusion over 10 min, followed by a 1-mg/min IV infusion

B. Patient's condition unstable

Consider immediate DC cardioversion or administration of an antiarrhythmic drug while correcting any electrolyte imbalance.

- Deliver a synchronized shock (360 J) (monophasic waveform) and repeat the synchronized shock as often as necessary at progressively increasing energy levels. In the conscious patient, premedicate the patient before cardioversion, using a sedative such as **midazolam** or **diazepam** as follows:
  - Midazolam 1 to 2 mg IV slowly over at least 2 min and repeat every 3 to 5 min, titrated to produce sedation/amnesia before cardioversion

OR

  Diazepam 5 to 15 mg with or without 2 to 5 mg **morphine** IV slowly to produce amnesia/analgesia before cardioversion
- Administer an antiarrhythmic drug such as **amiodarone.**
  - Amiodarone 150-mg IV infusion over 10 min, followed by a 1-mg/min IV infusion

VENTRICULAR TACHYCARDIA (VT), POLYMORPHIC (WITH PULSE) PROLONGED BASELINE QT INTERVAL TORSADE de POINTES (TdP) (WITH PULSE)

A. Patient's condition stable or unstable

◆ Consider a **magnesium sulfate** 1- to 2-g (8- to 16-mEq) IV bolus followed by a 20-mL flush of IV fluid if torsade de pointes or a hypomagnesic state is present. Follow with a maintenance IV infusion of 0.5 to 1.0 g (4 to 8 mEq) of magnesium sulfate to run for 1 h.

◆ Initiate transcutaneous overdrive pacing. If the patient has discomfort and is not hypotensive, administer a sedative such as **midazolam** or **diazepam** as follows:

◇ Midazolam 1 to 2 mg IV slowly over at least 2 min and repeat every 3 to 5 min, titrated to produce sedation/amnesia

OR

Diazepam 5 to 15 mg with or without 2 to 5 mg **morphine** IV slowly to produce amnesia/analgesia

AND

◆ Consider administration of one of the following **β-blockers** if not contraindicated and hypotension not present:

◇ **Esmolol** 0.5-mg/kg IV bolus over 1 min, followed by an IV infusion at a rate of 0.05 mg/kg/min and repeat the IV bolus twice, 5 min between each bolus, while increasing the rate of the IV infusion 0.05 mg/kg/min after each bolus. Then, if necessary, increase the IV infusion by 0.05 mg/kg/min every 5 min to a maximum of 0.30 mg/kg/min.

◇ **Atenolol** 5 mg IV over 5 min and repeat in 10 min for a total dose of 10 mg

◇ **Metoprolol** 5 mg IV over 2 to 5 min and repeat every 5 min up to a total dose of 15 mg

◆ Discontinue any antiarrhythmic agents that prolong the QT interval such as:

◇ Disopyramide

◇ Procainamide, quinidine, sotalol

◇ Any other agent that prolongs the QT interval (e.g., phenothiazines, tricyclic antidepressants)

AND

Correct any electrolyte imbalance.

◆ Deliver an unsynchronized shock (360 J) (monophasic waveform) and repeat the unsynchronized shock as often as necessary. In the conscious patient, if the patient's condition permits it, premedicate the patient before cardioversion, using a sedative such as **midazolam** or **diazepam** as follows:

◇ Midazolam 1 to 2 mg IV slowly over at least 2 min and repeat every 3 to 5 min, titrated to produce sedation/amnesia before cardioversion

OR

Diazepam 5 to 15 mg with or without 2 to 5 mg **morphine** IV slowly to produce amnesia/analgesia before cardioversion

PREMATURE ATRIAL CONTRACTIONS (PACs)
PREMATURE JUNCTIONAL CONTRACTIONS (PJCs)

A. Patient's condition stable or unstable

◆ Discontinue such drugs as:
  ◇ Stimulants
  ◇ Sympathomimetic drugs
  ◇ Digitalis, if digitalis toxicity is suspected

PREMATURE VENTRICULAR CONTRACTIONS (PVCs)

A. Patient's condition stable or unstable

◆ Consider one of the following drugs:
  ◇ A **β-blocker,** especially if PVCs are associated with an acute coronary syndrome
  ◇ Amiodarone
  ◇ Lidocaine

VENTRICULAR FIBRILLATION (VF)
PULSELESS VENTRICULAR TACHYCARDIA (VT)

- Assess airway, breathing and circulation
- Perform CPR
- Provide oxygen
- Attach monitor
- Check rhythm

- Give 1 shock at 360 J Monophasic (biphasic dose is device speific)

- Resume CPR for five cycles
- Check rhythm

- Give 1 shock at 360 J Monophasic (biphasic dose is device specific)
- Resume CPR
- Secure airway and confirm placement; limiting interruptions to CPR
- Establish IV/IO access; limiting interruptions to CPR

- Administer epinephrine 1 mg IV/IO; repeat every 3 to 5 minutes

  OR

  Administer vasopressin 40 U IV/IO; one time only

- Resume CPR for five cycles
- Check rhythm

- Give 1 shock at 360 J Monophasic (biphasic dose is device specfic)
- Resume CPR for five cycles

- Consider using antiarrhythmics:
  - Amiodarone (300 mg IV/IO once, repeat at 150 mg IV/IO)
  - Lidocaine (1.0 Give 1 shock 360 J Monophasic) (biphasic dose is device specfic)
    - 1.5 mg/kg for the first dose, 0.50-0.75 mg/kg IV for subsequent doses. Maximum dose of 3 mg/kg

VENTRICULAR ASYSTOLE

- Assess airway, breathing and circulation
- Perform CPR
- Provide oxygen

- Attach monitor
- Check rhythm
- Resume CPR for five cycles

- Secure airway and confirm placement; limiting interruptions to CPR
- Establish IV/IO access; limiting interruptions to CPR

- Administer epinephrine 1 mg IV/IO; repeat every 3 to 5 minutes

OR

Administer vasopressin 40 U IV/IO; one time only
- Consider atropine 1.0 mg IV/IO; repeat every 3-5 minutes (maximum dose 3 mg)
- Resume CPR for five cycles
- Check rhythm

- Search for and treat
  - Hypovolemia
  - Hypoxia
  - Hydrogen ion excess
  - Hypokalemia or hyperkalemia
  - Hypocalcemia
  - Toxic exposures
  - Cardiac tamponade
  - Tension pneumothorax
  - Coronary or pulmonary thrombosis
  - Trauma

PULSELESS ELECTRICAL ACTIVITY

- ◆ Assess airway, breathing and circulation
- ◆ Perform CPR
- ◆ Provide oxygen

- ◆ Attach monitor
- ◆ Check rhythm
- ◆ Resume CPR for five cycles

- ◆ Secure airway and confirm placement; limiting interruptions to CPR
- ◆ Establish IV/IO access; limiting interruptions to CPR

- ◆ Administer epinephrine 1 mg IV/IO; repeat every 3 to 5 minutes
  OR
  Administer vasopressin 40 U IV/IO; one time only
- ◆ Consider atropine 1.0 mg IV/IO; repeat every 3-5 minutes (maximum dose 3 mg)
- ◆ Resume CPR for five cycles
- ◆ Check rhythm

- ◆ Search for and treat
  - ◇ Hypovolemia
  - ◇ Hypoxia
  - ◇ Hydrogen ion excess
  - ◇ Hypokalemia or hyperkalemia
  - ◇ Hypocalcemia
  - ◇ Toxic exposures
  - ◇ Cardiac tamponade
  - ◇ Tension pneumothorax
  - ◇ Coronary or pulmonary thrombosis
  - ◇ Trauma

Bundle Branch and Fascicular Blocks

RIGHT BUNDLE BRANCH BLOCK (RBBB)

QRS Duration: ≥ 0.12 second in complete RBBB; 0.10 to 0.11 second in incomplete RBBB.

QRS Axis: Normal or right axis deviation ($+90°$ to $+110°$).

ST Segments: May be depressed in leads V_1-V_2.

T Waves: May be inverted in leads V_1-V_2.

QRS Complexes:
With an intact interventricular septum

Leads V_1 and V_2
Wide QRS with a classic triphasic rSR′ ("M" or "rabbit ears") pattern:
◆ Initial small r wave
◆ Deep, slurred S wave
◆ Late (terminal) tall R′ wave

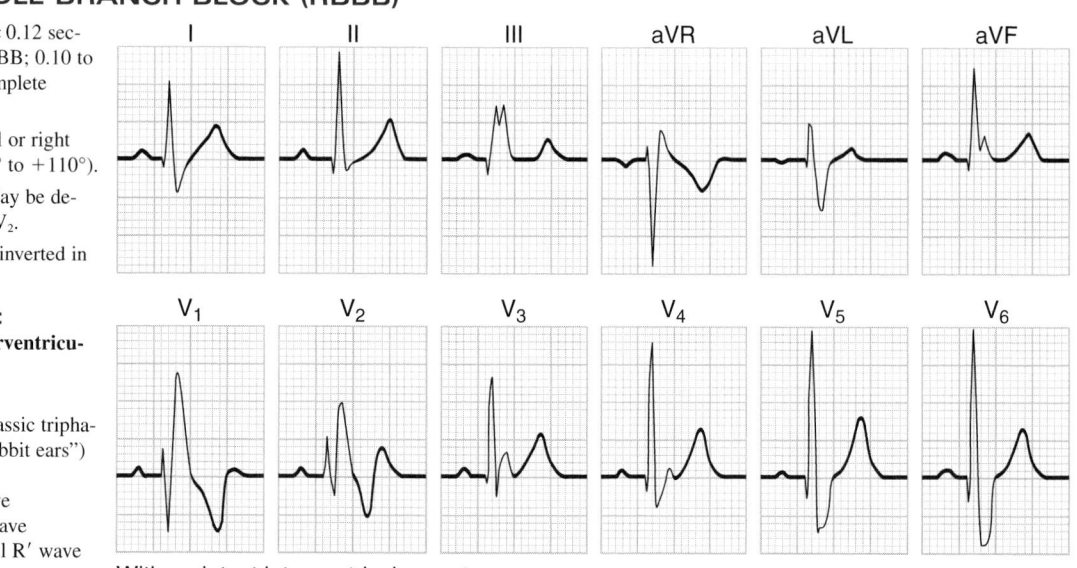

With an intact interventricular septum

Leads I, aVL, and V₅-V₆

Wide QRS with a typical qRS pattern:

- Initial small q wave
- Tall R wave
- Late (terminal) deep, slurred S wave

QRS Complexes:
Without an intact interventricular septum

Leads V₁ and V₂

Wide QRS with a QSR pattern:

- Absent initial small r wave
- Deep QS wave
- Late (terminal) tall R wave

Leads I, aVL, and V₅-V₆

Wide QRS with an RS pattern:

- Absent initial small q wave
- Tall R wave
- Late (terminal) deep, slurred S wave

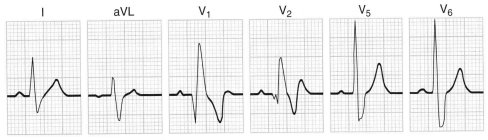

Without an intact interventricular septum

LEFT BUNDLE BRANCH BLOCK (LBBB)

QRS Duration: ≥0.12 second in complete LBBB; 0.10 to 0.11 second in incomplete LBBB.

QRS Axis: Commonly, left axis deviation (-30° to -90°), but may be normal.

ST Segments: Depressed in leads I, aVL, and V_5-V_6; elevated in leads V_1-V_3.

T Waves: Inverted in leads I, aVL, and V_5-V_6; elevated in leads V_1-V_3.

QRS Complexes:

With an intact interventricular septum

Leads V_1-V_3

Wide QRS with an rS or QS pattern:

- Initial small r wave
- Deep, wide S wave

OR

- Absent R wave
- Deep, wide QS wave

Leads I, aVL, and V_5-V_6

Wide QRS with an R pattern:

- Absent initial small q wave
- Tall, wide, slurred R wave with or without notching, and a prolonged VAT

With an intact interventricular septum

QRS Complexes:
Without an intact interventricular septum

Leads V₁ and V₂

Wide QRS with an rS pattern:

♦ Small narrow r wave

♦ Deep, wide S wave

Leads I, aVL, and V₅-V₆

Wide QRS with a qR pattern:

♦ Small q wave

♦ Tall, wide, slurred R wave with or without notching, and a prolonged VAT

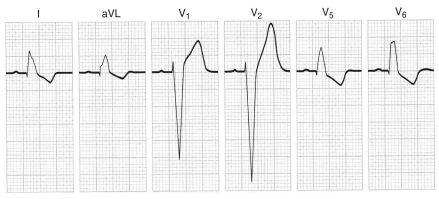

Without an intact interventricular septum

LEFT ANTERIOR FASCICULAR BLOCK (LAFB)

QRS Duration: Normal, <0.10 second.

QRS Axis: Left axis deviation ($-30°$ to $-90°$).

ST Segments: Normal.

T Waves: Normal.

QRS Complexes:

Leads I and aVL
Narrow QRS:
◆ Initial small q wave

Leads II, III, and aVF
Narrow QRS:
◆ Initial small r wave
◆ Deep S wave, typically larger than the R wave

QRS Pattern: A typical q_1r_3 pattern is present.

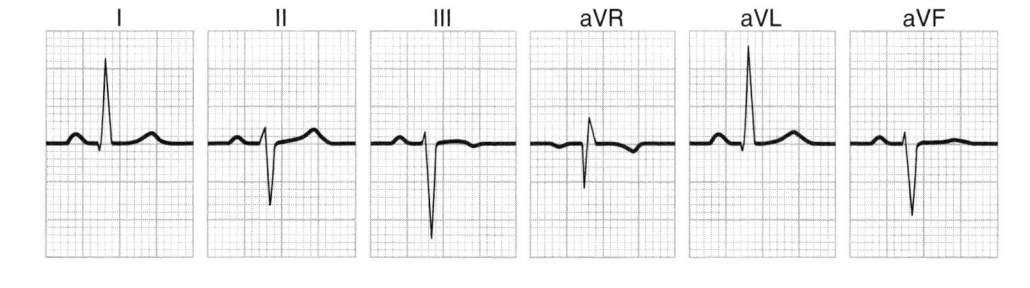

LEFT POSTERIOR FASCICULAR BLOCK (LPFB)

QRS Duration: Normal, <0.10 second.

QRS Axis: Right axis deviation (+110° to +180°).

ST Segments: Normal.

T Waves: Normal.

QRS Complexes:

Leads I, aVL, and V_5-V_6

Narrow QRS:

♦ Absent q wave in leads I, aVL, and V_5-V_6

♦ Initial small r wave in leads I and aVL

♦ Deep S wave in leads I and aVL

Leads II, III, and aVF

Narrow QRS:

♦ Initial small q wave

♦ Tall R wave

QRS Pattern: A typical q_3r_1 pattern is present.

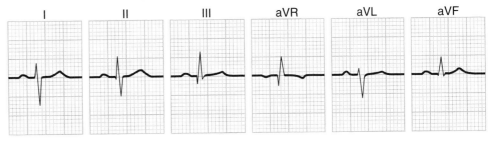

Miscellaneous ECG Changes

CHAMBER ENLARGEMENT

RIGHT ATRIAL ENLARGEMENT

P Waves

Duration: Usually normal (0.10 second or less).

Shape: Typically tall and symmetrically peaked P waves in leads II, III, and aVF—the **P pulmonale.** Sharply peaked biphasic P waves in lead V_1-V_2.

Direction: Positive (upright) in leads II, III, and aVF; biphasic in V_1-V_2 with the initial deflection greater than the terminal deflection.

Amplitude: 2.5 mm or greater in leads II, III, and aVF.

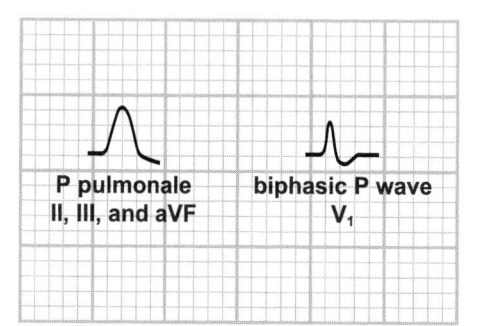

P pulmonale
II, III, and aVF

biphasic P wave
V_1

LEFT ATRIAL ENLARGEMENT

P Waves

Duration: Usually greater than 0.10 second.

Shape:

- A broad positive (upright) P wave, 0.12 second or greater in duration, in any lead.
- A wide, notched P wave with two "humps" 0.04 second or more apart—the **P mitrale,** usually present in leads I, II, and V_4-V_6. The first hump represents the depolarization of the right atrium; the second hump represents the depolarization of the enlarged left atrium.
- A biphasic P wave, greater than 0.10 second in total duration, with the terminal, negative component 1 mm (0.10 mV) or more deep and 1 mm (0.04 second) or more in duration (i.e., 1 small square or greater) commonly present in leads V_1-V_2. The initial, positive (upright) component of the P wave represents the depolarization of the right atrium; the terminal, negative component represents the depolarization of the enlarged left atrium.

Direction: Positive (upright) in leads I, II, and V_4-V_6 and biphasic in leads V_1-V_2; may be negative in leads III and aVF.

Amplitude: Usually normal (0.5 to 2.5 mm).

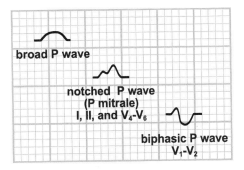

broad P wave

notched P wave
(P mitrale)
I, II, and V_4-V_6

biphasic P wave
V_1-V_2

RIGHT VENTRICULAR HYPERTROPHY (RVH)

P Waves: Right atrial enlargement usually present.

QRS Complexes

Duration: Normal, 0.10 second or less.

Ventricular Activation Time (VAT): Prolonged beyond the upper normal limit of 0.035 second in leads V_1-V_2.

Q Waves: May be present in leads II, III, and aVF.

R Waves: Tall R waves in leads II, III, and V_1. Usually 7 mm or more (>0.7 mV) in height and equal to or greater than the S waves in depth in lead V_1. Relatively tall R waves also in leads V_2-V_3.

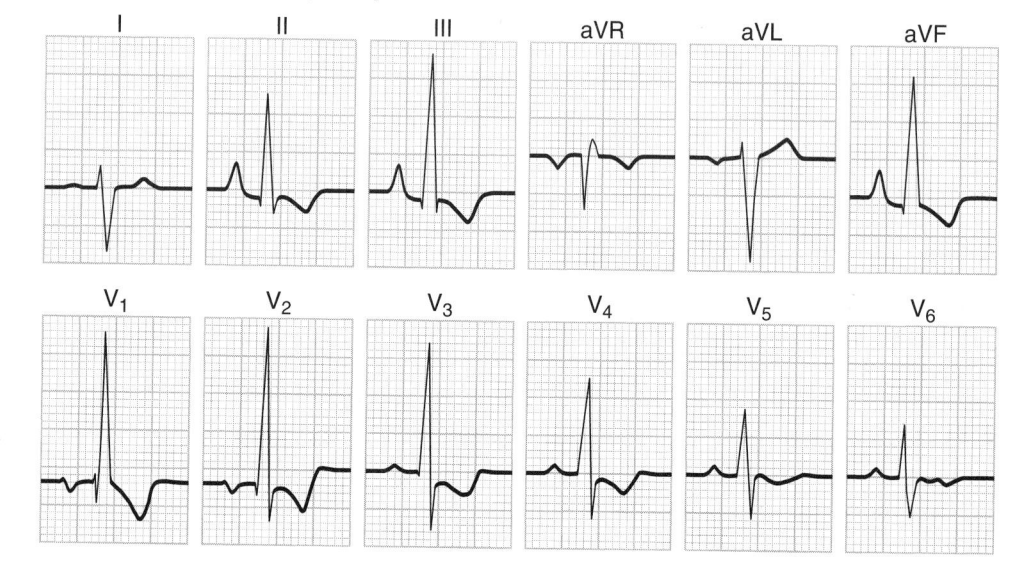

Note: Tall R waves equal to or greater than the S waves in lead V_1 may also be present in acute posterior myocardial infarction (MI) and in counterclockwise rotation of the heart.

S Waves: Relatively deeper than normal in leads I and V_4-V_6. In lead V_6, the depth of the S waves may be greater than the height of the R waves.

ST Segments: "Downsloping" ST segment depression of 1 mm or more may be present in leads II, III, aVF, and V_1 and sometimes in leads V_2 and V_3.

T Waves: Often inverted in leads II, III, aVF, and V_1 and sometimes in leads V_2 and V_3.

Note: The downsloping ST segment depression and the T wave inversion together form the "strain" pattern characteristic of longstanding RVH, giving the so-called "hockey stick" appearance to the QRS-ST-T complex.

QRS Axis: Right axis deviation of $+90°$ or more; $\geq +110°$ in adults; $\geq +120°$ in the young.

LEFT VENTRICULAR HYPERTROPHY (LVH)

P Waves: Left atrial enlargement usually present.

QRS Complexes

  Duration: Normal, 0.10 second or less.

  Ventricular Activation Time (VAT): Prolonged beyond the upper normal limit to 0.05 second or more in leads V_5 and V_6.

  R Waves: Tall R waves in leads I, aVL, and V_5-V_6.

  S Waves: Deep S waves in leads III and V_1-V_2.

  QRS Axis: Usually normal, but may be left axis deviation ($> -30°$).

ST Segments: "Downsloping" ST segment depression of 1 mm or more in leads I, aVL, and V_5-V_6.

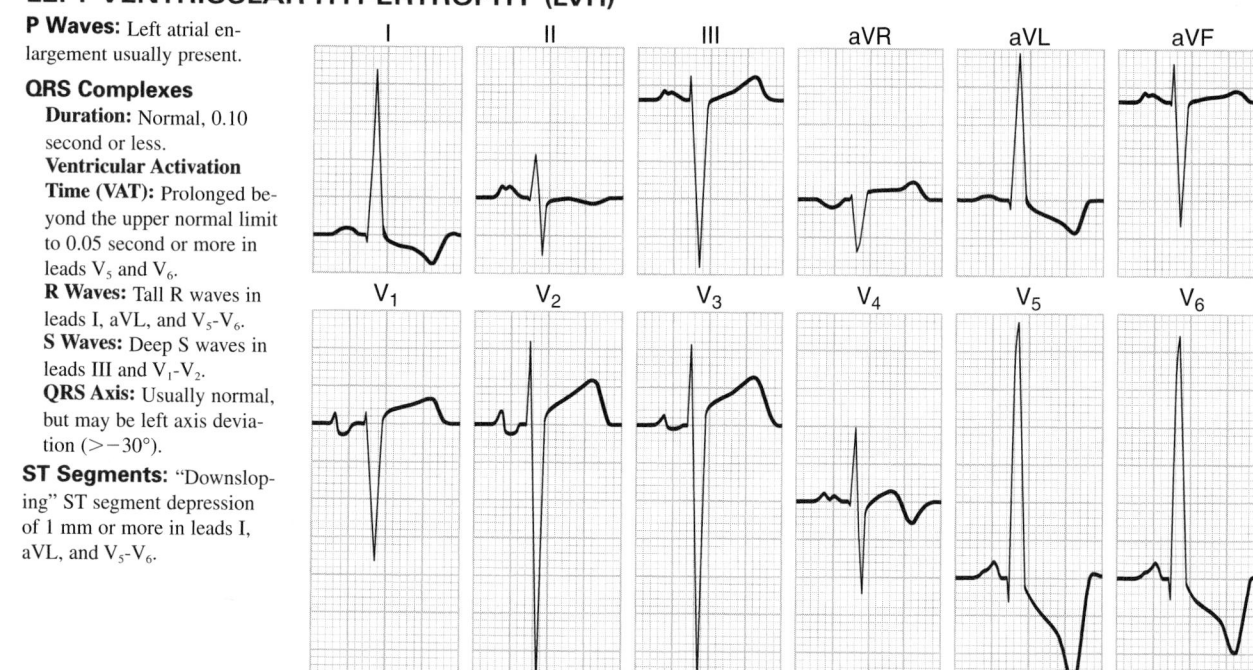

T Waves: Inverted in leads I, aVL, and V_5-V_6. The inverted T waves together with the "downsloping" ST segment depression form the "strain" pattern characteristic of longstanding LVH—the so-called "hockey stick" appearance of the QRS-ST-T complex.

Diagnosis of LVH: The amplitude (or voltage) of the R waves and the depth (or voltage) of the S waves considered to indicate LVH in certain leads are shown in the following table.

| Wave | Lead | | | | |
	I	III	aVL	V_1 or V_2	V_5 or V_6
R	≥20 mm (≥2.0 mV)		≥11 mm (≥1.1 mV)		≥30 mm (≥3.0 mV)
S		≥20 mm (≥2.0 mV)		≥30 mm (≥3.0 mV)	

Sum of R and S Waves: The sum of the amplitude of the R waves and the depth of the S waves (in mm or mV) in certain leads with the most prominent R and S waves is diagnostic of LVH if it equals or exceeds the following values:

$$R \text{ (I, II, or III)} + S \text{ (I, II, or III)} = ≥20 \text{ mm } (≥2.0 \text{ mV})$$

$$R \text{ I} + S \text{ III} = ≥25 \text{ mm } (≥2.5 \text{ mV})$$

$$S V_1 \text{ (or } S V_2) + R V_5 \text{ (or } R V_6) = ≥35 \text{ mm } (≥3.5 \text{ mV})$$

Criteria Diagnostic of LVH: LVH is present if criteria 1 and 2 are met:

Criteria 1

$$R \text{ I or } S \text{ III} = ≥20 \text{ mm } (≥2.0 \text{ mV})$$

OR

$$R \text{ I} + S \text{ III} = ≥25 \text{ mm } (≥2.5 \text{ mV})$$

OR

$$S V_1 \text{ (or } S V_2) + R V_5 \text{ (or } R V_6) = ≥35 \text{ mm } (≥3.5 \text{ mV})$$

Criteria 2

QRS axis between $-15°$ and $-30°$ or greater than $-30°$ (left axis deviation)

OR

ST segment depression of ≥1mm in leads with an R wave having the amplitude (or voltage) criteria of left ventricular hypertrophy (see table at left).

QT Intervals: Normal.

PERICARDITIS

QRS Complexes

Amplitude: Normal if pleural effusion absent. QRS complexes may be low in voltage (amplitude) if pleural effusion is present. If pleural effusion is severe, cardiac tamponade may occur, causing the QRS complexes to alternate between normal and low voltage, coincident with respiration (electrical alternans).

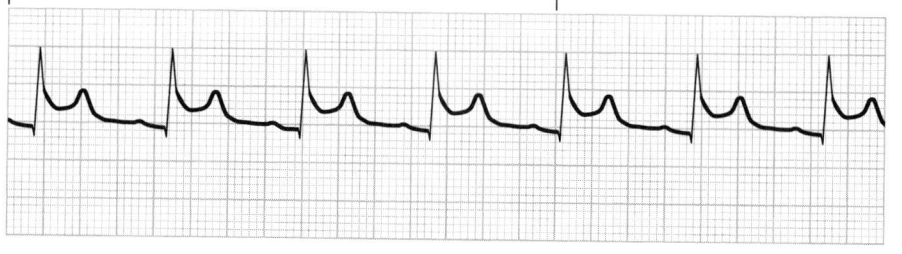

Abnormal Q waves/QS complexes: Absent.

ST Segments: Elevated (concave elevation) in acute phase of pericarditis in the ECG leads overlying the affected pericardium (see table). Reciprocal ST segment depression is usually not present. The ST segment is either normal or depressed in aVR. The ST segments return to normal as the pericarditis resolves.

T Waves: Elevated during the acute phase of pericarditis in the leads with ST segment elevation. The elevated T waves become inverted as the pericarditis resolves.

Location of Pericarditis	Leads With ST Segment Elevation
Anterior	V_2-V_4
Lateral	I, aVL, V_5-V_6
Inferior	II, III, aVF
Generalized	I, II, III, aVL, aVF, V_2-V_6

ELECTROLYTE IMBALANCE

HYPERKALEMIA

P Waves: Begin to flatten out and become wider at a serum potassium level of about 6.5 mEq/L and disappear at levels of about 7.0-9.0 mEq/L.

PR Intervals: May be normal or prolonged, greater than 0.20 second. Absent when the P waves disappear.

QRS Complexes: Begin to widen at serum potassium levels of about 6.0-6.5 mEq/L, becoming markedly slurred and abnormally widened beyond 0.12 second at 10 mEq/L. At this point they "merge" with the following T waves, resulting in a "sine wave" QRS-ST-T pattern.

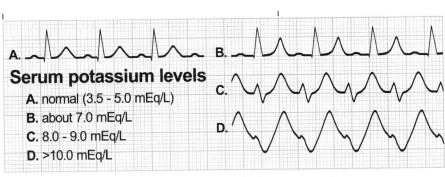

ST Segments: Disappear at a serum potassium level of about 6 mEq/L.

T Waves: Become typically tall and peaked with a narrower than normal base at serum potassium levels of about 5.5-6.5 mEq/L. Earliest T wave changes best seen in leads II, III, and V_2-V_6.

Associated Arrhythmias

- Sinus arrest (may occur at a serum potassium level of about 7.5 mEq/L)
- Cardiac standstill (may occur at serum potassium levels of about 10 to 12 mEq/L)
- Ventricular fibrillation (may occur at serum potassium levels of about 10 to 12 mEq/L)

HYPOKALEMIA

P Waves: Become typically tall and symmetrically peaked, with an amplitude of ≥2.5 mm in leads II, III, and aVF at a serum potassium level of ≤2 mEq/L (pseudo P pulmonale).

QRS Complexes: Begin to widen at a serum potassium level of about 3.0 mEq/L.

ST Segments: May become depressed by 1 mm or more.

T Waves: Begin to flatten at a serum potassium level of about 3.0 mEq/L and continue to become smaller as the U waves increase in size.

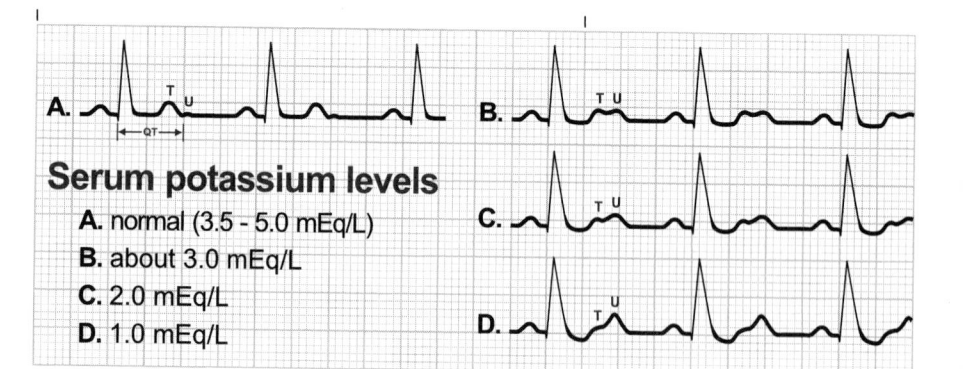

Serum potassium levels

A. normal (3.5 - 5.0 mEq/L)
B. about 3.0 mEq/L
C. 2.0 mEq/L
D. 1.0 mEq/L

The T waves may either merge with the U waves or become inverted.

U Waves: Begin to increase in size, becoming as tall as the T waves (i.e., "prominent") at a serum potassium level of about 3.0 mEq/L and, at about 2 mEq/L, becoming taller than the T waves. The U waves reach "giant" size and fuse with the T waves at 1 mEq/L.

QT Intervals: May appear to be prolonged when the U waves become prominent and fuse with the T waves but actually remain normal.

Associated Arrhythmias: Ventricular arrhythmias, including torsade de pointes (may occur in hypokalemia in the presence of digitalis).

HYPERCALCEMIA

QT Intervals: Shorter than normal for the heart rate.

HYPOCALCEMIA

ST Segments: Prolonged.

QT Intervals: Prolonged beyond the normal limits for the heart rate because of the prolonged ST segments.

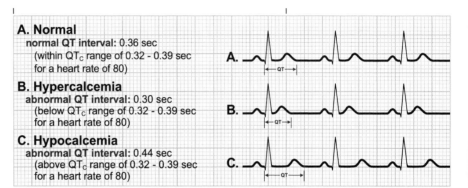

A. Normal
  normal QT interval: 0.36 sec
    (within QT_C range of 0.32 - 0.39 sec
    for a heart rate of 80)

B. Hypercalcemia
  abnormal QT interval: 0.30 sec
    (below QT_C range of 0.32 - 0.39 sec
    for a heart rate of 80)

C. Hypocalcemia
  abnormal QT interval: 0.44 sec
    (above QT_C range of 0.32 - 0.39 sec
    for a heart rate of 80)

Serum calcium levels
A. Normal (2.1-2.6 mEq/L)
B. Hypercalcemia (>2.6 mEq/L)
C. Hypocalcemia (<2.1 mEq/L)

DRUG EFFECT

DIGITALIS

PR Intervals: Prolonged over 0.2 second.

ST Segments: Depressed 1 mm or more in many of the leads, with a characteristic "scooped-out" appearance.

T Waves: May be flattened, inverted, or biphasic.

QT Intervals: Shorter than normal for the heart rate.

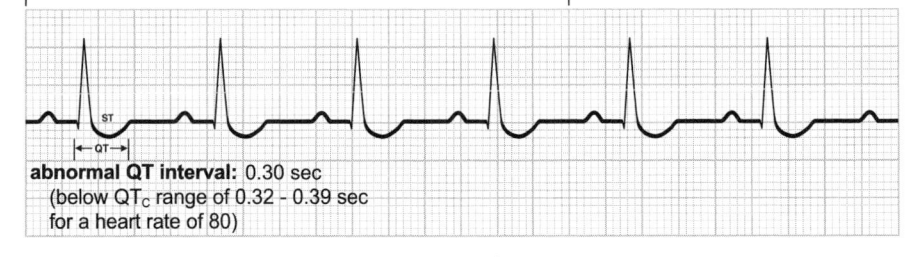

abnormal QT interval: 0.30 sec (below QT$_C$ range of 0.32 - 0.39 sec for a heart rate of 80)

Effects of Digitalis Toxicity: Excessive administration of digitalis may cause the following excitatory and inhibitory effects on the heart and its electrical conduction system.

Excitatory effects include the following:
- Premature atrial contractions
- Atrial tachycardia with or without block
- Nonparoxysmal junctional tachycardia
- Premature ventricular contractions
- Ventricular tachycardia
- Ventricular fibrillation

Inhibitory effects include the following:
- Sinus bradycardia
- Sinoatrial (SA) exit block
- Atrioventricular (AV) block

PROCAINAMIDE

PR Intervals: May be prolonged.

QRS Complexes

Duration: May be increased beyond 0.12 second, a sign of procainamide toxicity.

R waves: May be decreased in amplitude.

ST Segments: May be depressed 1 mm or more.

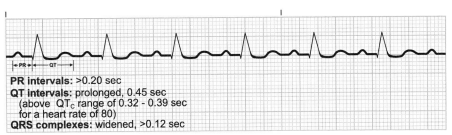

PR intervals: >0.20 sec
QT intervals: prolonged, 0.45 sec
(above QT$_c$ range of 0.32 - 0.39 sec for a heart rate of 80)
QRS complexes: widened, >0.12 sec

T Waves: May be decreased in amplitude, and occasionally widened and notched because of the appearance of a U wave.

QT Intervals: May occasionally be prolonged beyond the normal limits for the heart rate, a sign of procainamide toxicity.

Effects of Procainamide Toxicity: Excessive administration of procainamide may cause the following excitatory and inhibitory effects on the heart and its electrical conduction system.

Excitatory effects include the following:

◆ Premature ventricular contractions

◆ Torsade de pointes (occurrence less common than in quinidine toxicity)

◆ Ventricular fibrillation

Inhibitory effects include the following:

◆ Depression of myocardial contractility, which may cause hypotension and congestive heart failure

◆ Atrioventricular (AV) block

◆ Ventricular asystole

QUINIDINE

P Waves: May be wide, often notched.

PR Intervals: May be prolonged beyond normal.

QRS Complexes

Duration: May be increased beyond 0.12 second, a sign of quinidine toxicity.

ST Segments: May be depressed 1 mm or more.

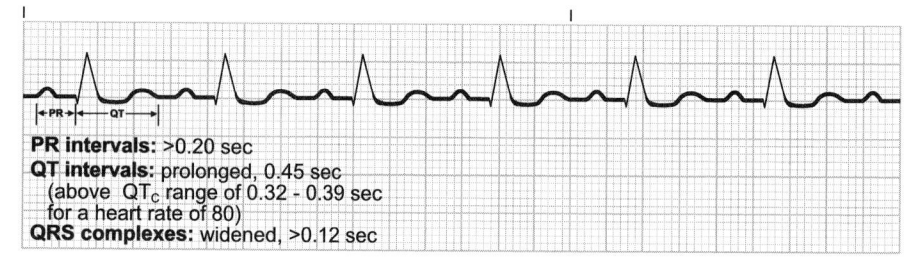

PR intervals: >0.20 sec
QT intervals: prolonged, 0.45 sec
    (above QT$_c$ range of 0.32 - 0.39 sec
    for a heart rate of 80)
QRS complexes: widened, >0.12 sec

T Waves: May be decreased in amplitude, wide, and notched, or they may be inverted. The notching is caused by the appearance of a U wave as the T wave widens.

QT Intervals: May be prolonged beyond the normal limits for the heart rate. Prolongation of the QT interval is a sign of quinidine toxicity.

Effects of Quinidine Toxicity: Excessive administration of quinidine may cause the following excitatory and inhibitory effects on the heart and its electrical conduction system.

Excitatory effects include the following:
◆ Premature ventricular contractions
◆ Torsade de pointes (occurrence more common than in procainamide toxicity)
◆ Ventricular fibrillation

Inhibitory effects include the following:
◆ Depression of myocardial contractility, which may cause hypotension and congestive heart failure
◆ Sinoatrial (SA) exit block
◆ Atrioventricular (AV) block
◆ Ventricular asystole

PULMONARY DISEASE

CHRONIC OBSTRUCTIVE PULMONARY DISEASE (COPD)

P Waves: Right atrial enlargement may be present (P pulmonale).

QRS Complexes: Usually of low voltage. Poor R-wave progression across the precordium is usually present.

QRS Axis: May be greater than +90°.

Associated Arrhythmias:
- Premature atrial contractions
- Wandering atrial pacemaker
- Multifocal atrial tachycardia
- Atrial flutter
- Atrial fibrillation

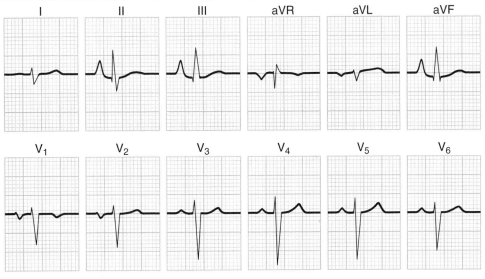

PULMONARY EMBOLISM (ACUTE)

P Waves: Right atrial enlargement may be present (P pulmonale).

QRS Complexes
Q Waves: Abnormal Q waves in lead III.
S Waves: Deep S waves in lead I.
T Waves: Inverted T waves in lead III.

ST Segments/T Waves: Right ventricular "strain" pattern may be present in leads V_1-V_3.

QRS Pattern: An $S_1Q_3T_3$ pattern may occur acutely. In addition, a right bundle branch block may also occur.

QRS Axis: Greater than +90°.

Associated Arrhythmias: Sinus tachycardia.

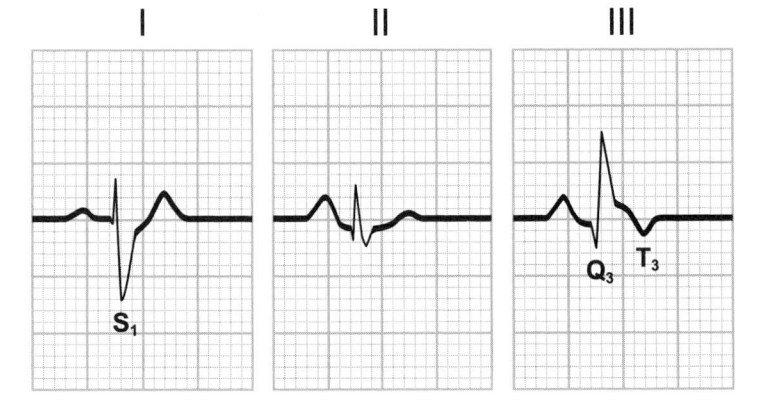

CHRONIC COR PULMONALE

P Waves: Right atrial enlargement present (P pulmonale).

QRS Complexes: Right ventricular hypertrophy present.

ST Segments/T Waves: Right ventricular "strain" pattern in leads V_1-V_3.

QRS Axis: Greater than +90°.

Associated Arrhythmias

- Premature atrial contractions
- Wandering atrial pacemaker
- Multifocal atrial tachycardia
- Atrial flutter
- Atrial fibrillation

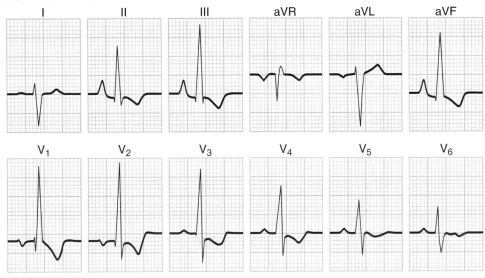

EARLY REPOLARIZATION

QRS Complexes: Abnormal Q waves usually absent.

ST Segments: Elevated by about 1 to 3 mm or more in leads I, II, and aVF and the precordial leads V_2-V_6. May be depressed in lead aVR.

T Waves: Usually normal.

Lead II

HYPOTHERMIA

PR Intervals: May occasionally be prolonged, greater than 0.20 second.

QRS Complexes: May occasionally be abnormally wide, greater than 0.12 second. Typically followed by an Osborn wave.

QT Intervals: Corrected QT interval (QTc interval) may be occasionally prolonged.

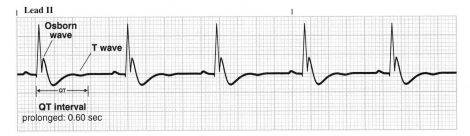

Lead II

Osborn wave

T wave

QT

QT interval prolonged: 0.60 sec

Osborn Wave: A narrow positive deflection at the junction of the QRS complex and the ST segment. Typically seen in the leads facing the left ventricle (leads I, II, III, aVL, aVF, and V_3-V_6).

Associated Arrhythmias

- ◆ Sinus bradycardia
- ◆ Junctional arrhythmias
- ◆ Ventricular arrhythmia

PREEXCITATION SYNDROMES

VENTRICULAR PREEXCITATION

PR Intervals: Abnormally short, usually less than 0.12 second; between 0.09 and 0.12 second.

QRS Complexes: Duration greater than 0.10 second. A delta wave is present.

ATRIO-HIS PREEXCITATION

PR Intervals: Abnormally short, usually less than 0.12 second.

QRS Complexes: Duration normal, 0.10 second or less.

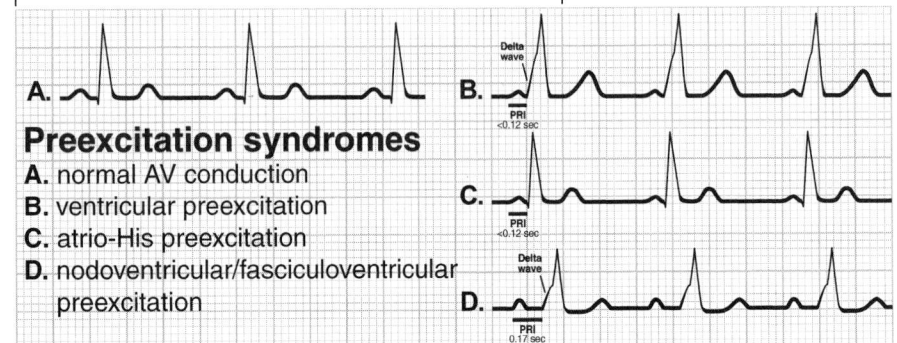

Preexcitation syndromes

A. normal AV conduction
B. ventricular preexcitation
C. atrio-His preexcitation
D. nodoventricular/fasciculoventricular preexcitation

NODOVENTRICULAR/FASCICULOVEN-TRICULAR PREEXCITATION

PR Intervals: Normal, 0.12 second or greater.

QRS Complexes: Duration greater than 0.10 second. A delta wave is present.

CAUSES OF THE HEART CHAMBER ENLARGEMENTS, ELECTROLYTE IMBALANCES, AND MISCELLANEOUS CONDITIONS RESPONSIBLE FOR THE ECG CHANGES PRESENTED IN SECTION IV

Cause of Right Atrial Enlargement (Right Atrial Dilatation and Hypertrophy): Increased pressure and/or volume in the right atrium (i.e., right atrial overload), commonly the result of the following:

♦ Pulmonary valve stenosis
♦ Tricuspid valve stenosis and insufficiency (relatively rare)
♦ Pulmonary hypertension from various causes, including chronic obstructive pulmonary disease (COPD), status asthmaticus, pulmonary embolism, pulmonary edema, mitral valve stenosis or insufficiency, and congenital heart disease

The result of right atrial enlargement is, typically, a tall, symmetrically peaked P wave—the **P pulmonale.**

Cause of RVH: Increased pressure and/or volume in the right ventricle (i.e., right ventricular overload), commonly the result of the following:

♦ Pulmonary valve stenosis and other congenital heart defects (e.g., atrial and ventricular septal defects)
♦ Tricuspid valve insufficiency (relatively rare)

♦ Pulmonary hypertension from various causes, including chronic obstructive pulmonary disease (COPD), status asthmaticus, pulmonary embolism, pulmonary edema, and mitral valve stenosis or insufficiency

Cause of Left Atrial Enlargement (Left Atrial Dilatation and Hypertrophy): Increased pressure and/or volume in the left atrium (i.e., left atrial overload), commonly the result of the following:

♦ Mitral valve stenosis and insufficiency
♦ Acute MI
♦ Left heart failure
♦ Left ventricular hypertrophy from various causes, such as aortic stenosis or insufficiency, systemic hypertension, and hypertrophic cardiomyopathy

The result of left atrial enlargement is, typically, a wide, notched P wave—the **P mitrale.** Such P waves may also result from a delay or block of the progression of the electrical impulses through the interatrial conduction tract between the right and left atria.

Cause of LVH: Increased pressure and/or volume in the left ventricle (i.e., left ventricular overload), commonly the result of the following:
♦ Mitral insufficiency
♦ Aortic stenosis or insufficiency
♦ Systemic hypertension
♦ Acute MI
♦ Hypertrophic cardiomyopathy

Cause of Hyperkalemia: Excess of serum potassium above the normal levels of 3.5-5.0 mEq/L. The most common causes of hyperkalemia are the following:
♦ Kidney failure
♦ Certain diuretics (e.g., triamterene)

Cause of Hypokalemia: Deficiency of serum potassium below the normal levels of 3.5-5.0 mEq/L. Causes of hypokalemia are the following:
♦ Loss of potassium in body fluids through vomiting, gastric suction, and excessive use of diuretics (the most common causes)
♦ Low serum magnesium levels (hypomagnesemia)
  The ECG characteristics of hypomagnesemia, incidentally, resemble those of hypokalemia.

Cause of Hypercalcemia: Excess of serum calcium above the normal levels of 2.1-2.6 mEq/L (or 4.25-5.25 mg/100 mL). Common causes of hypercalcemia include the following:
♦ Adrenal insufficiency
♦ Hyperparathyroidism
♦ Immobilization
♦ Kidney failure
♦ Malignancy
♦ Sarcoidosis
♦ Thyrotoxicosis
♦ Vitamin A and D intoxication

Cause of Hypocalcemia: Deficiency of serum calcium below the normal levels of 2.1-2.6 mEq/L (or 4.25-5.25 mg/100 mL). Common causes of hypocalcemia include the following:
♦ Chronic steatorrhea
♦ Diuretics (such as furosemide or ethacrynic acid)
♦ Respiratory alkalosis and hyperventilation
♦ Osteomalacia in adults and rickets in children
♦ Pregnancy
♦ Hypoparathyroidism
♦ Hypomagnesemia (possibly because of release of parathyroid hormone)

Cause of Early Repolarization: A normal ECG variant that occurs in normal healthy people, commonly in young persons and sometimes in the elderly.

Cause of Hypothermia: A drop of the core body temperature to ≤95° F.

Cause of Preexcitation Syndromes

- **Ventricular Preexcitation.** Aberrant conduction of an electrical impulse through an abnormal accessory AV pathway that bypasses the AV junction, resulting in premature depolarization of the ventricles and an abnormally short PR interval.

- **Atrio-His Preexcitation.** Aberrant conduction of an electrical impulse through abnormal atrio-His fibers that bypass the AV node, resulting in an abnormally short PR interval but normal depolarization of the ventricles.

- **Nodoventricular/Fasciculoventricular Preexcitation.** Aberrant conduction of an electrical impulse through abnormal nodoventricular or fasciculoventricular fibers that bypass the entire bundle of His or the distal part of it, respectively, resulting in premature depolarization of the ventricles and a normal PR interval.

Acute Myocardial Infarction

LOCATIONS OF MYOCARDIAL INFARCTION

Septal MI	**Localized anterior MI**	**Anteroseptal MI**	**Lateral MI**

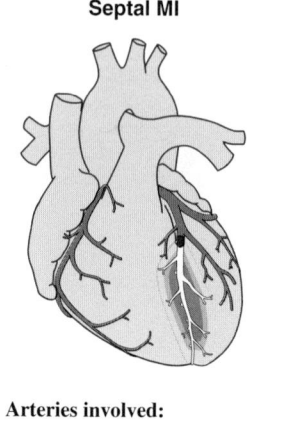 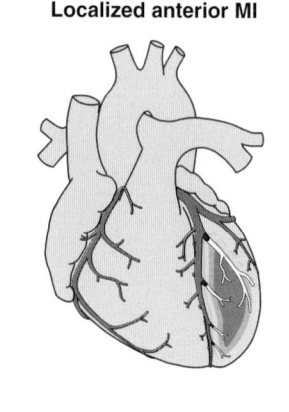 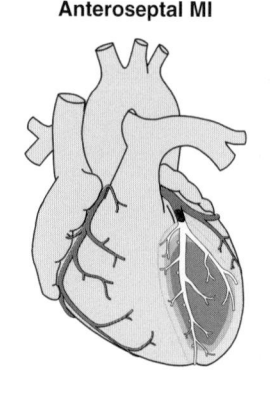 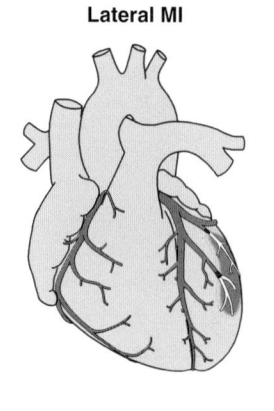

Arteries involved:

Left anterior descending artery
　Septal perforator branches

Left anterior descending artery
　Diagonal branches

Left anterior descending artery
　Septal perforating branches
　Diagonal branches

Left anterior descending artery
　Diagonal branches
Left circumflex artery
　Anterolateral marginal branch

Anterolateral MI	**Extensive anterior MI**	**Inferior MI**	**Posterior MI**	**Right ventricular MI**

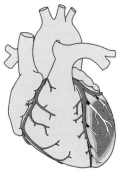 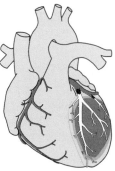 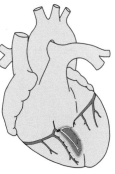 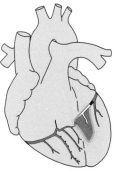 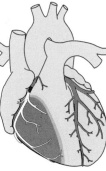

Arteries involved:

Left anterior descending
  artery
  Diagonal branches
Left circumflex artery
  Anterolateral marginal
  branch

Left anterior descending
  artery
Left circumflex artery
  Anterolateral marginal
  branch

Right coronary (or left
circumflex) artery
  Posterior left ventric-
  ular branches

Distal left circumflex
artery and/or its posterolateral branch

Right coronary artery

SEPTAL MYOCARDIAL INFARCTION

Early

Phase 1: First Few Hours (0 to 2 Hours)

ECG Changes

In facing leads V_1-V_2:

◆ Absence of normal "septal" r waves in leads V_1-V_2, resulting in QS waves in these leads

◆ ST segment elevation with tall T waves in leads V_1-V_2

In leads I, II, III, aVF, and V_4-V_6:

◆ Absence of normal "septal" q waves where normally present in leads I, II, III, aVF, and V_4-V_6

In opposite leads II, III, and aVF:

◆ No significant ECG changes in leads II, III, and aVF

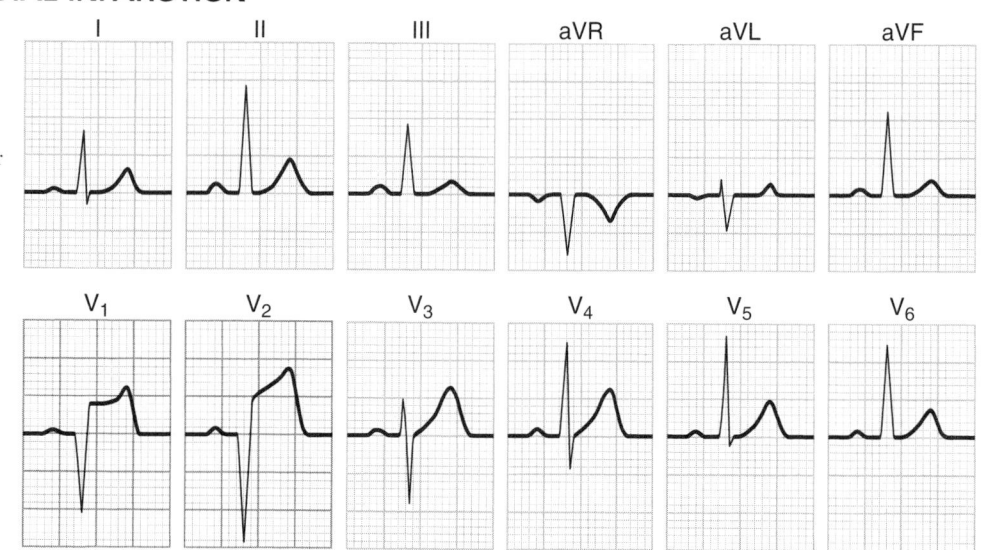

Phase 2: First Day (2 to 24 Hours)

ECG Changes

In facing leads V_1-V_2:

- Maximal ST segment elevation in leads V_1-V_2

Late

Phase 3: Second and Third Day (24 to 72 Hours)

ECG Changes

In facing leads V_1-V_2:

- QS complexes with T wave inversion in leads V_1-V_2
- Return of ST segments to baseline in leads V_1-V_2

In opposite leads II, III, and aVF:

- No significant ECG changes in leads II, III, and aVF

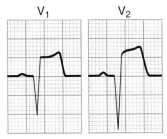

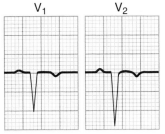

ANTERIOR (LOCALIZED) MYOCARDIAL INFARCTION

Early

**Phase 1: First Few Hours
(0 to 2 Hours)**

ECG Changes

In facing leads V_3-V_4:

◆ ST segment elevation with
tall T waves and taller than
normal R waves in leads
V_3-V_4

In opposite leads II, III, and
aVF:

◆ No significant ECG changes
in leads II, III, and aVF

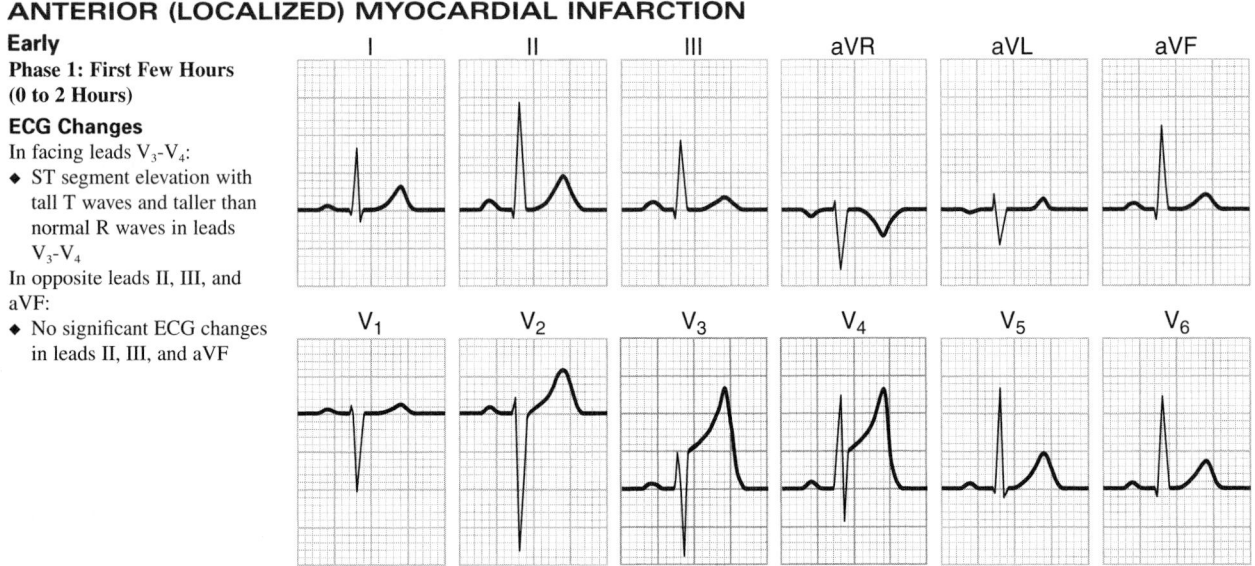

Phase 2: First Day (2 to 24 Hours)

ECG Changes

In facing leads V_3-V_4:

- ◆ Minimally abnormal Q waves in leads V_3-V_4
- ◆ Maximal ST segment elevation in leads V_3-V_4

Late

Phase 3: Second and Third Day (24 to 72 Hours)

ECG Changes

In facing leads V_3-V_4:

- ◆ QS complexes with T wave inversion in leads V_3-V_4
- ◆ Return of ST segments to baseline in leads V_3-V_4

In opposite leads II, III, and aVF:

- ◆ No significant ECG changes in leads II, III, and aVF

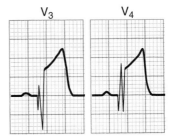

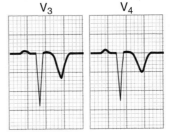

ANTEROSEPTAL MYOCARDIAL INFARCTION

Early
Phase 1: First Few Hours
(0 to 2 Hours)

ECG Changes

In facing leads V_1-V_4:

♦ Absence of normal "septal" r waves in leads V_1-V_2, resulting in QS waves in these leads

♦ ST segment elevation with tall T waves in leads V_1-V_4

♦ Taller than normal R waves in leads V_3-V_4

In leads I, II, III, aVF, and V_4-V_6:

♦ Absence of normal "septal" q waves where normally present in leads I, II, III, aVF, and V_4-V_6

In opposite leads II, III, and aVF:

♦ No significant ECG changes in leads II, III, and aVF

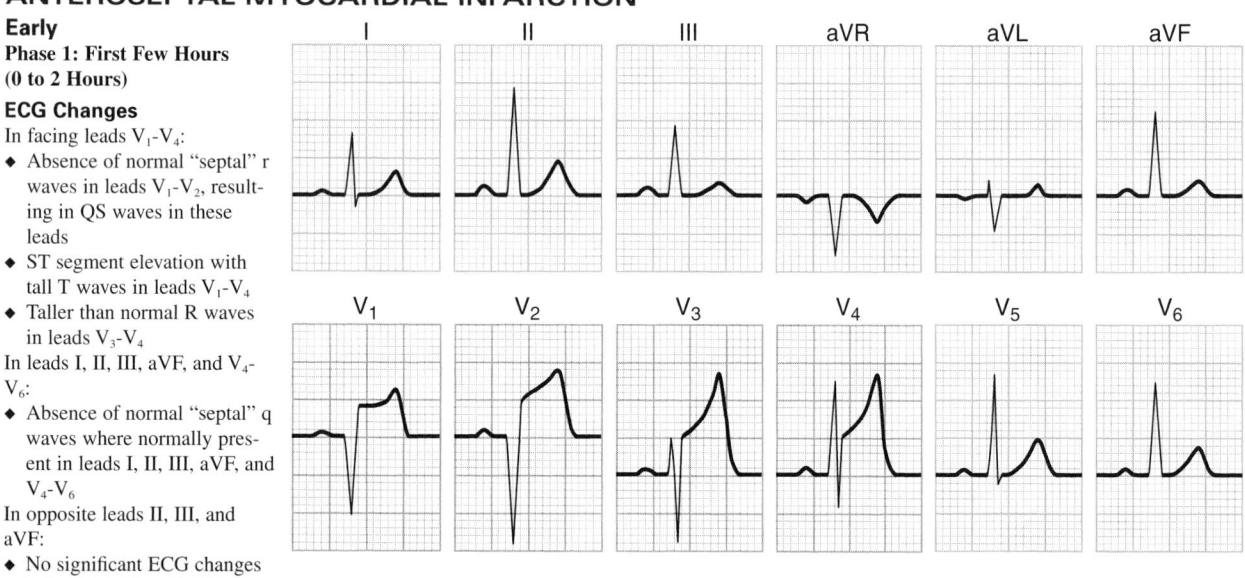

Phase 2: First Day (2 to 24 Hours)

ECG Changes

In facing leads V_1-V_4:

- Minimally abnormal Q waves in leads V_3-V_4
- Maximal ST segment elevation in leads V_1-V_4

Late

Phase 3: Second and Third Day (24 to 72 Hours)

ECG Changes

In facing leads V_1-V_4:

- QS complexes with T wave inversion in leads V_1-V_4
- Return of ST segments to baseline in leads V_1-V_4

In opposite leads II, III, and aVF:

- No significant ECG changes in leads II, III, and aVF

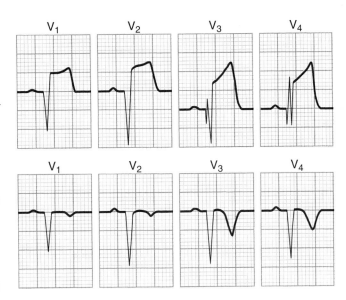

LATERAL MYOCARDIAL INFARCTION

Early
Phase 1: First Few Hours (0 to 2 Hours)

ECG Changes

In facing leads I, aVL, and V_5-V_6:

♦ ST segment elevation with tall T waves and taller than normal R waves in leads I, aVL, and lead V_5 or V_6 or both

In opposite leads II, III, and aVF:

♦ ST segment depression in leads II, III, and aVF

Phase 2: First Day (2 to 24 Hours)

ECG Changes

In facing leads I, aVL, and V_5-V_6:

♦ Minimally abnormal Q waves in leads I and aVL and lead V_5 or V_6 or both

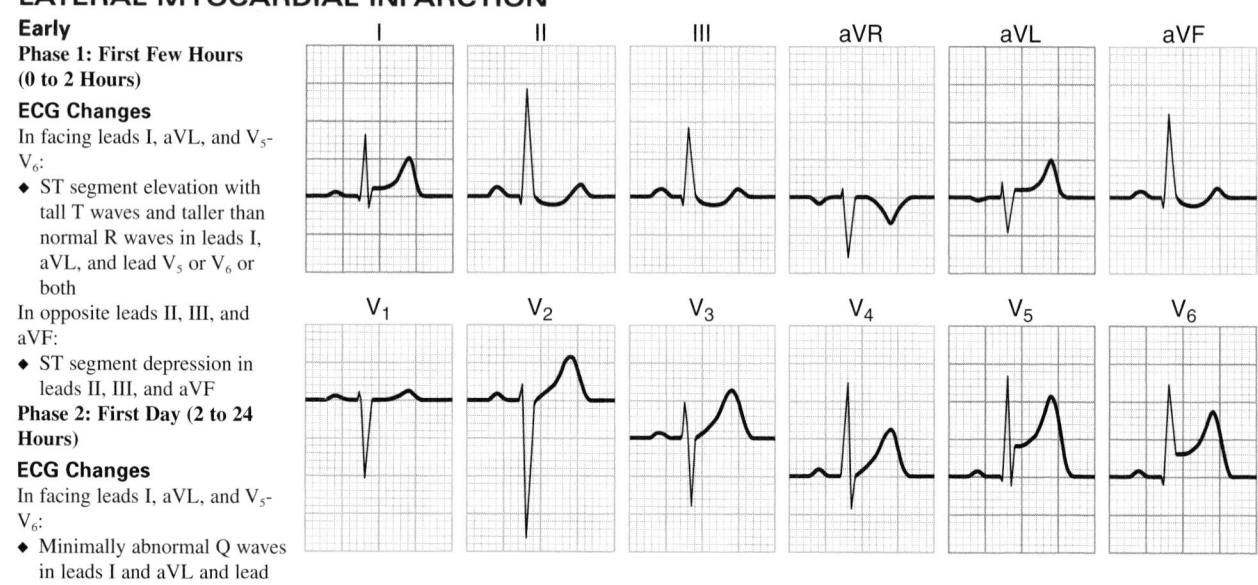

- Maximal ST segment elevation in leads I and aVL and lead V_5 or V_6 or both

Late
Phase 3: Second and Third Day (24 to 72 Hours)
ECG Changes
In facing leads I, aVL, and V_5-V_6:

- Abnormal Q waves and small R waves with T wave inversion in leads I and aVL
- QS waves or complexes and decreased or absent R waves with T wave inversion in lead V_5 or V_6 or both
- Return of ST segments to baseline

In opposite leads II, III, and aVF:

- Tall T waves in leads II, III, and aVF
- Return of ST segments to baseline

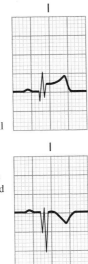

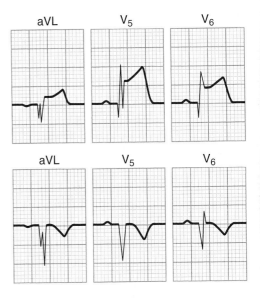

ANTEROLATERAL MYOCARDIAL INFARCTION

Early

Phase 1: First Few Hours (0 to 2 Hours)

ECG Changes

In facing leads I, aVL, and V_3-V_6:

♦ ST segment elevation with tall T waves and taller than normal R waves in leads I, aVL, and V_3-V_6

In opposite leads II, III, and aVF:

♦ ST segment depression in leads II, III, and aVF

Phase 2: First Day (2 to 24 Hours)

ECG Changes

In facing leads I, aVL, and V_3-V_6:

♦ Minimally abnormal Q waves in leads I, aVL, and V_3-V_6

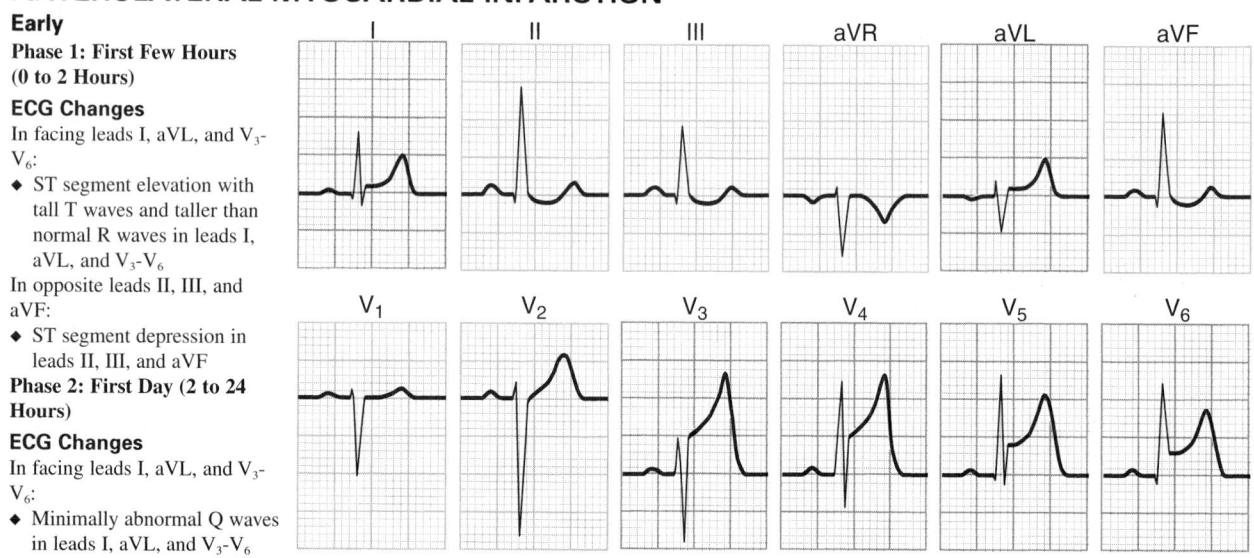

- Maximal ST segment elevation in leads I, aVL, and V₃-V₆

Late

Phase 3: Second and Third Day (24 to 72 Hours)

ECG Changes

In facing leads I, aVL, and V₃-V₆:

- Abnormal Q waves and small R waves with T wave inversion in leads I and aVL
- QS waves or complexes and decreased or absent R waves with T wave inversion in leads V₃-V₆
- Return of ST segments to baseline

In opposite leads II, III, and aVF:

- Tall T waves in leads II, III, and aVF
- Return of ST segments to baseline

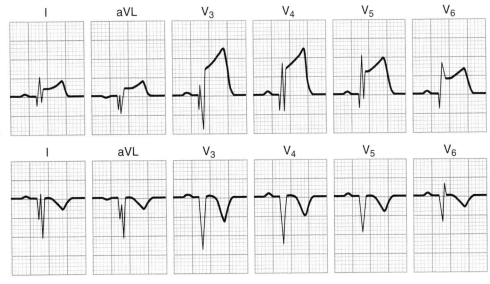

EXTENSIVE ANTERIOR MYOCARDIAL INFARCTION

Early

**Phase 1: First Few Hours
(0 to 2 Hours)**

ECG Changes

In facing leads I, aVL, and V_1-V_6:

♦ Absence of normal "septal" r waves in leads V_1-V_2, resulting in QS complexes in these leads

♦ ST segment elevation with tall T waves in leads I, aVL, and V_1-V_6

♦ Taller than normal R waves in leads I, aVL, and V_3-V_6

In leads I, II, III, aVF, and V_4-V_6:

♦ Absence of normal "septal" q waves where normally present in leads I, II, III, aVF, and V_4-V_6

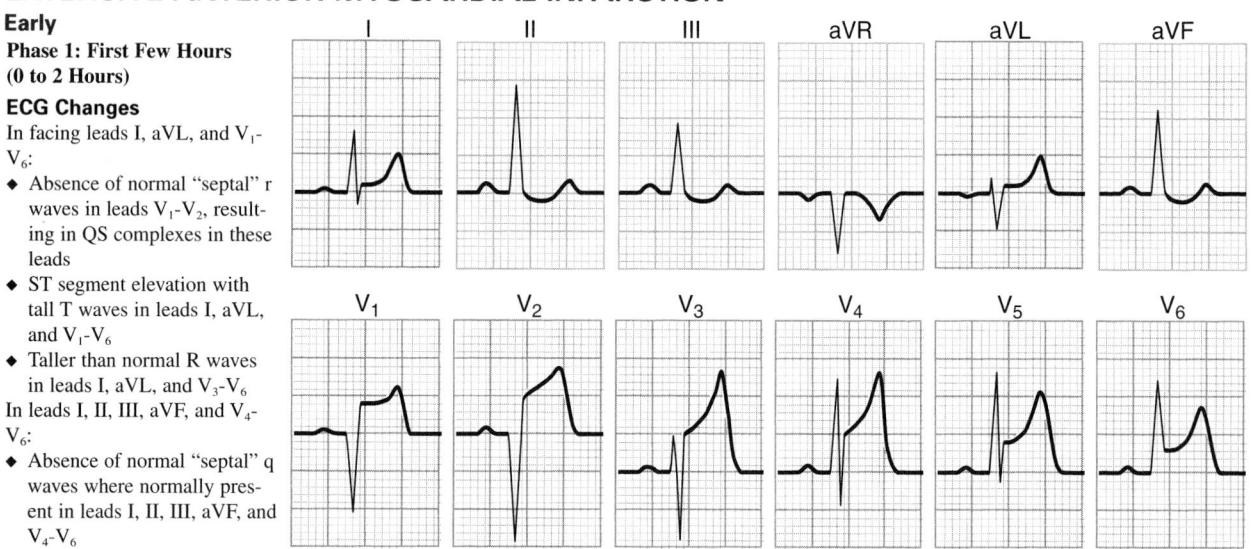

In opposite leads II, III, and aVF:

♦ ST segment depression in leads II, III, and aVF

Phase 2: First Day (2 to 24 Hours)

ECG Changes

In facing leads I, aVL, and V₁-V₆:

♦ Minimally abnormal Q waves in leads I, aVL, and V₃-V₆

♦ Maximal ST segment elevation in leads I, aVL, and V₁-V₆

Late

Phase 3: Second and Third Day (24 to 72 Hours)

ECG Changes

In facing leads I, aVL, and V₁-V₆:

♦ Abnormal Q waves and small R waves with T wave inversion in leads I and aVL

♦ QS waves or complexes with T wave inversion in leads V₁-V₅ and sometimes V₆

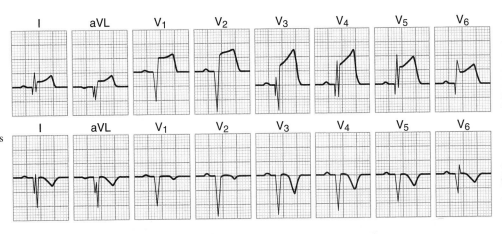

♦ R waves absent in V₁-V₂ and decreased or absent in V₃-V₅ and sometimes V₆

♦ Return of ST segments to baseline

In opposite leads II, III, and aVF:

♦ Tall T waves in leads II, III, and aVF

♦ Return of ST segments to baseline

INFERIOR MYOCARDIAL INFARCTION

Early

**Phase 1: First Few Hours
(0 to 2 Hours)**

ECG Changes

In facing leads II, III, and aVF:

♦ ST segment elevation with tall T waves and taller than normal R waves in leads II, III, and aVF

In opposite leads I and aVL:

♦ ST segment depression in leads I and aVL

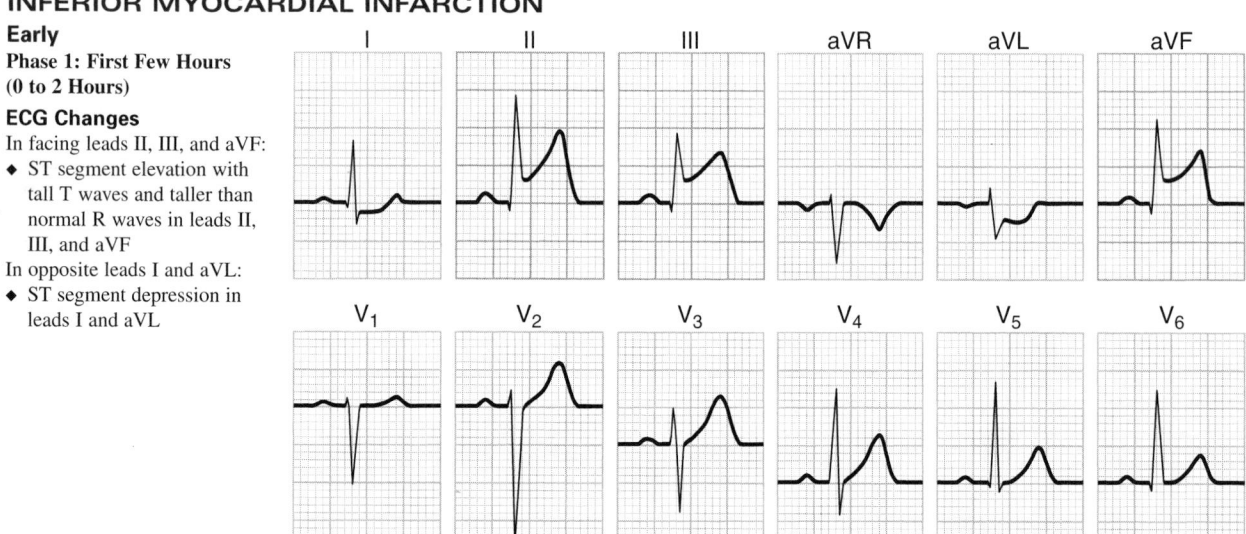

Phase 2: First Day (2 to 24 Hours)

ECG Changes

In facing leads II, III, and aVF:

- ◆ Minimally abnormal Q waves in leads II, III, and aVF
- ◆ Maximal ST segment elevation in leads II, III, and aVF

Late

Phase 3: Second and Third Day (24 to 72 Hours)

ECG Changes

In facing leads II, III, and aVF:

- ◆ QS waves or complexes and decreased or absent R waves with T wave inversion in leads II, III, and aVF
- ◆ Return of ST segments to baseline

In opposite leads I and aVL:

- ◆ Tall T waves in leads I and aVL
- ◆ Return of ST segments to baseline

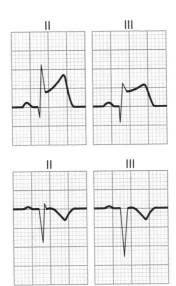

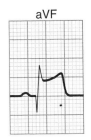

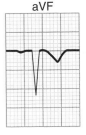

POSTERIOR MYOCARDIAL INFARCTION

Early

Phase 1: First Few Hours (0 to 2 Hours)

ECG Changes

In facing leads: No facing leads present.

In opposite leads V_1-V_4:

◆ ST segment depression in leads V_1-V_4

◆ T wave inversion in V_1 and sometimes V_2

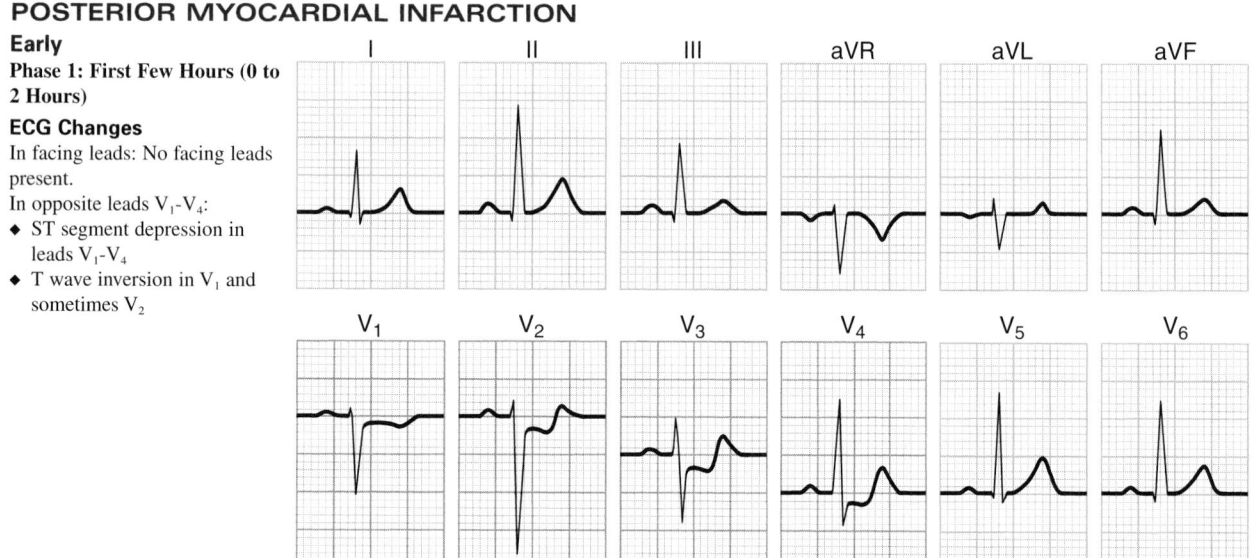

Phase 2: First Day (2 to 24 Hours)

ECG Changes

In facing leads: No facing leads present.

In opposite leads V_1-V_4:

♦ Maximal ST segment depression in leads V_1-V_4

Late

Phase 3: Second and Third Day (24 to 72 Hours)

ECG Changes

In facing leads: No facing leads present.

In opposite leads V_1-V_4:

♦ Large R waves with tall T waves in leads V_1-V_4; the R waves in lead V_1 are tall and wide ($\geq$0.04 sec in width) with slurring and notching

♦ Smaller than normal S waves in lead V_1, resulting in an R/S ratio of $\geq$1 in this lead

♦ Return of ST segments to baseline in leads V_1-V_4

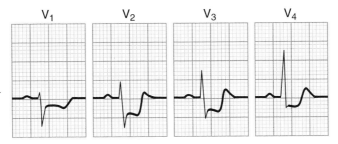

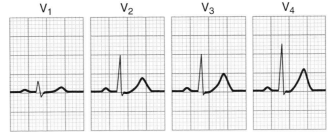

RIGHT VENTRICULAR MYOCARDIAL INFARCTION

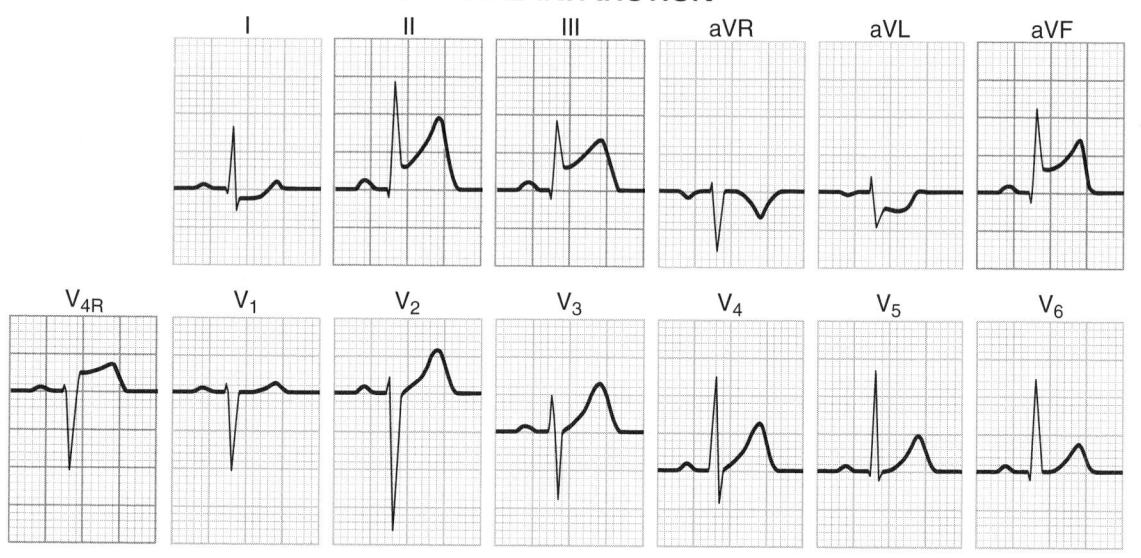

Early

Phase 1: First Few Hours (0 to 2 Hours)

ECG Changes

In facing leads II, III, aVF, and V_{4R}:

- ST segment elevation in leads II, III, aVF, and V_{4R}
- Tall T waves and taller than normal R waves in leads II, III, and aVF

In opposite leads I and aVL:

- ST segment depression in leads I and aVL

Phase 2: First Day (2 to 24 Hours)

ECG Changes

In facing leads II, III, aVF, and V_{4R}:

- Minimally abnormal Q waves in leads II, III, and aVF
- Maximal ST segment elevation in leads II, III, and aVF
- ST segment elevation in lead V_{4R}, but ST segment may be normal

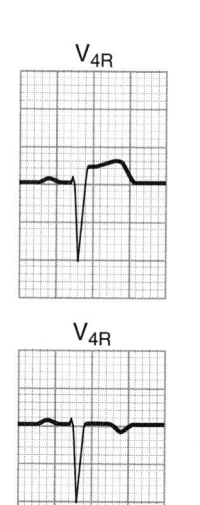
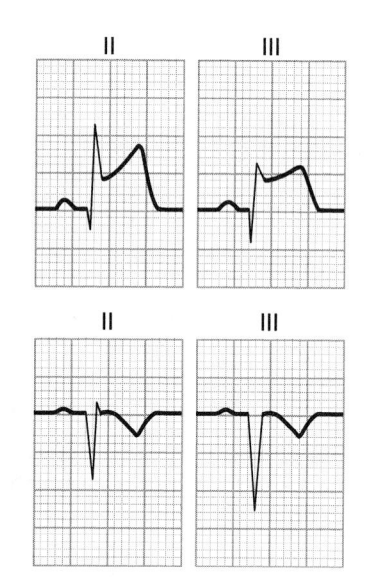
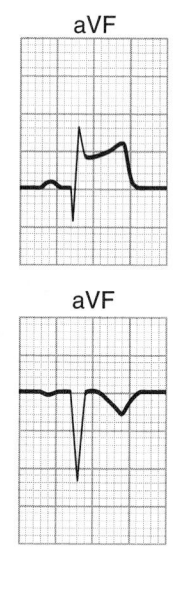

V4R II III aVF

V4R II III aVF

Late
Phase 3: Second and Third Day (24 to 72 Hours)
ECG Changes
In facing leads II, III, aVF, and V_{4R}:

♦ QS waves or complexes and decreased or absent R waves in leads II, III, and aVF

♦ T wave inversion in leads II, III, aVF, and V_{4R}

♦ Return of ST segments to baseline

In opposite leads I and aVL:

♦ Tall T waves in leads I and aVL

♦ Return of ST segments to baseline

Management of Acute Myocardial Infarction

SIGNS AND SYMPTOMS OF ACUTE MYOCARDIAL INFARCTION

Pain is the most common symptom of acute myocardial infarction (MI), appearing in 70% to 80% of the patients with acute MI who are not in shock or cardiac arrest. One or more of the following signs and symptoms frequently accompany the pain of acute MI, depending on the degree of mechanical pump failure present and whether an arrhythmia is present. It is important to note that many of these signs and symptoms may be present even in the absence of pain, as in a so-called *silent acute MI*. The finding of any one or more of the following symptoms should lead one to suspect acute MI, especially if the patient is middle-aged or older.

Symptoms in Acute Myocardial Infarction

◆ **General and neurological symptoms.** Anxiety and apprehension, extreme fatigue and weakness, restlessness, and agitation with a fear of impending death (or a sense of impending doom) are common. Lightheadedness or dizziness, confusion, disorientation, drowsiness, or loss of consciousness may also be present.

◆ **Cardiovascular.** Chest pain and palpitations or "skipping of the heart" are usually present in the majority of the patients.

◆ **Respiratory.** Dyspnea is common, often accompanied by a sensation of suffocation; a tight, constricted feeling in the chest; and even pain on breathing. Wheezing; spasmodic coughing, often productive of copious, frothy sputum, frequently pink- or blood-tinged (hemoptysis); and choking may be present.

◆ **Gastrointestinal.** Nausea with or without vomiting and a loss of appetite (anorexia) are common. If gastrointestinal symptoms are present and, especially, if the chest pain radiates to the epigastrium, the patient often misinterprets the symptoms as being those of indigestion and ignores them. Thirst and an urge to defecate may also be present.

Signs in Acute Myocardial Infarction

◆ **General appearance and neurological signs.** The patient may be alert and oriented initially but restless, anxious, and apprehensive or confused and disoriented. The patient may become drowsy and unresponsive and then lose consciousness and convulse.

◆ **Vital Signs**

  ◇ **Pulse.** The pulse is usually rapid, over 100/min (tachycardia), but may be 60 to 100/min (normal) or less than 60/min (bradycardia). The rhythm may be regular or irregular. The force of the pulse may be normal, strong and full, or if hypotension or shock is present, weak and thready.

  ◇ **Respirations.** The respirations are typically greater than 16/min (tachypnea) and shallow, but may be 12 to 16/min (normal, eupnea) or less. The rhythm of the respirations may be regular or irregular; their depth may be normal, shallow, or deep. The respirations may be labored and noisy or gasping. Hyperpnea may be present. The accessory muscles of respiration may be prominent during breathing if severe pulmonary congestion and edema are present.

⬧ **Blood pressure.** The systolic blood pressure may be normal, elevated (above 140 mm Hg), or low (less than 90 mm Hg) if hypotension or shock is present.

◆ **Skin.** The skin is usually pale, cold, sweaty, and clammy. Often cyanosis of the skin, fingernail beds, and mucous membranes is present because of pulmonary congestion and edema. The skin is mottled and bluish-red if shock is present. The lips may be normal in color, pale, or cyanotic.

◆ **Eyes.** The eyes appear normal, or if hypotension or shock is present they may be glassy, with a lackluster and vacant, dull stare or a ground-glass appearance. They may have an apprehensive and fearful look. The eyelids may be drooping. The pupils may be normal or dilated.

◆ **Veins.** The neck veins with the patient lying flat or propped up at a 45-degree angle may be normal, moderately distended (in left heart failure and mild right heart failure), markedly distended and pulsating (in severe right heart failure), or collapsed (in hypotension or shock). The superficial veins of the body may be normal, distended, or collapsed.

◆ **Cardiovascular.** The heart sounds are usually distant. A fourth heart sound (S_4) in late diastole and often a systolic murmur are present. If left heart failure complicates acute MI, a third heart sound (S_3) appears early in diastole. A gallop rhythm exists when a third or fourth heart sound or both are present.

◆ **Respiratory.** Breathing may be normal or labored and noisy. Wheezing, dry coarse rattling in the throat, spasmodic coughing with expectoration of frothy sputum, often pink- or blood-tinged (hemoptysis); and choking may be present. Dullness to percussion may be present over one or both lungs, particularly at the bases of the lungs posteriorly. On auscultation, the breath sounds may be normal, decreased, or absent. Rales, wheezes, rhonchi, and possibly loud gurgling or bubbling sounds may be present at one or both bases of the lungs only or up to the scapulae posteriorly or throughout the lungs.

◆ **Body tissue edema.** Pitting edema in the lower extremities, particularly in the ankles and feet and in front of the tibia (pedal and pretibial edema), lower part of the back over the spine (presacral edema), and abdominal wall may be present in right heart failure. If the tissues of the entire body are edematous, anasarca is present.

◆ **Abdomen.** The liver and spleen may be engorged with fluid and swollen (hepatomegaly and splenomegaly) and painful to palpation in severe right heart failure. The abdominal cavity may also be distended with fluid (ascites) in right heart failure.

◆ **Arrhythmias.** An arrhythmia may be present.

ACUTE MYOCARDIAL INFARCTION MANAGEMENT

A. INITIAL ASSESSMENT AND MANAGEMENT OF A PATIENT WITH CHEST PAIN

Prehospital/Emergency Department
◆ Perform an initial assessment
  ◇ Establish and maintain an open airway
  ◇ Assess the ventilatory status
  ◇ Start monitoring the blood oxygen saturation
  ◇ Assess the circulatory status and level of consciousness
  ◇ Obtain the vital signs
◆ Administer high-concentration oxygen
◆ Start an IV drip of 500 mL of D_5W
◆ Start ECG monitoring

AND

Obtain a 12-lead ECG (plus lead V_{4R}, if indicated)
◆ Obtain a brief history and physical examination
If the chest pain is suggestive of an acute MI:
◆ Obtain blood samples for determination of serum cardiac markers, C-reactive protein, etc.
◆ Determine the patient's eligibility for reperfusion therapy using the thrombolytic therapy eligibility checklist, p.129

◆ Proceed to section B, *Initial Treatment and Assessment of Suspected Acute Myocardial Infarction.*

B. INITIAL TREATMENT AND ASSESSMENT OF SUSPECTED ACUTE MYOCARDIAL INFARCTION

Prehospital/Emergency Department
1. Initial treatment
◆ Administer a **chewable aspirin** 160 to 325 mg
If chest pain is present and the patient is not hypotensive and right ventricular MI is not suspected:
◆ Administer a **nitroglycerin** 0.4-mg sublingual tablet or lingual aerosol and repeat every 5 min twice

AND

If nitroglycerin is not effective after the third dose or the pain is severe:
◆ Administer **morphine sulfate** 1 to 3 mg IV slowly and repeat every 5 to 30 min up to a total dose of 25 to 30 mg
If the patient is apprehensive/anxious:
◆ Administer **diazepam** 5 to 15 mg IV slowly

If the patient is nauseous/vomiting:

- Administer **promethazine hydrochloride** 12.5 to 25 mg IV

2. ECG evaluation

If any of the following ECG changes are present, the ECG is diagnostic of an acute MI:

- ST-segment elevation of ≥1 mm in two or more contiguous leads (indicative of an acute anterior, lateral, inferior, or right ventricular MI)
- ST-segment depression of ≥1 mm in two or more contiguous precordial leads (indicative of an acute posterior MI)
- New or presumably new LBBB

3. Adjunctive treatment

If the ECG is diagnostic of an acute MI:

- Administer one of the following **ß-blockers** if not contraindicated and a right ventricular MI is not present:
  - ⬦ **Atenolol** 5 mg IV over 5 min and repeat in 10 min for a total dose of 10 mg

OR

  Metoprolol 5 mg IV over 2 to 5 min and repeat every 5 min to a total dose of 15 mg

- Consider the administration of **nitroglycerin** intravenously if *chest pain* continues or recurs or *hypertension, congestive heart failure,* or an *extensive anterior MI* is present (and the patient is not hypotensive and right ventricular MI not present):
  - ⬦ Nitroglycerin 12.5- to 25.0-μg IV bolus, followed by an IV infusion at a rate of 10 to 20 μg/min initially, then increasing the rate by 5 to 10 μg/min every 5 to 10 min if necessary until:
    - The chest pain or the symptoms of congestive heart failure are relieved
    - The mean arterial blood pressure drops by 10% in a normotensive patient
    - The mean arterial blood pressure drops by 30% in a hypertensive patient
    - The heart rate increases by 10 beats per minute, or
    - The maximum infusion rate of 200 μg/min is reached

AND

    If the mean arterial blood pressure drops below 80 mm Hg or the systolic blood pressure drops below 90 mm Hg at any time:
    - Slow or temporarily stop the IV infusion of nitroglycerin.

- Proceed to section C, *Reperfusion therapy* if acute MI is confirmed, and to the following as appropriate:
  - ⬦ Section II, *Arrhythmia Management*
  - ⬦ Section D, *Management of Congestive Heart Failure*
  - ⬦ Section E, *Management of Cardiogenic Shock*

C. REPERFUSION THERAPY
Prehospital/Emergency Department

If there are no contraindications to reperfusion therapy and the symptoms are of less than 12 hours duration:

◆ Administer one of the following **thrombolytic agents:**
  ◇ **Reteplase** 10-U IV bolus in 2 min; repeat in 30 min

OR

  Tenecteplase 30- to 50-mg IV bolus in 5 sec based on the patient's weight

NOTE: If a GP IIb/IIIa receptor inhibitor is administered in combination with a thrombolytic agent, reduce the thrombolytic agent's usual dosage in half.

AND

Administer an anticoagulant such as **low-molecular-weight (LMW) heparin** (enoxaparin) or **unfractionated heparin.**

  ◇ Enoxaparin 30-mg IV bolus, followed in 15 min by 1 mg/kg subcutaneously

OR

Unfractionated heparin 60-U/kg IV bolus (maximum 4000 U for patients ≥68 kg), followed by an IV infusion at a rate of 12-U/kg/hr to maintain an aPTT of 50 to 70 sec

◆ Consider the administration of one of the following platelet **GP IIb/IIIa receptor inhibitors:**
  ◇ **Abciximab** 0.25-mg/kg IV bolus, followed by an IV infusion at a rate of 0.125 μg/kg/min

OR

  Eptifibatide 180-μg/kg IV bolus, followed by an IV infusion at a rate of 2 μg/kg/min

Caution: Following the administration of any of the above, closely monitor the patient for any bleeding.

◆ With or without prior thrombolytic therapy, evaluate the patient for need of percutaneous coronary intervention (PCI)—coronary artery angioplasty and/or stenting.

Tenecteplase Dosage Table

Patient weight (kg)	<60 kg	60 to <70 kg	70 to <80 kg	80 to <90 kg	≥90 kg
TNK-tPA (mg)	30 mg	35 mg	40 mg	45 mg	50 mg
Volume (mL)	(6 mL)	(7 mL)	(8 mL)	(9 mL)	(10 mL)

D. MANAGEMENT OF CONGESTIVE HEART FAILURE

Left Heart Failure Secondary to Left Ventricular Myocardial Infarction

Prehospital/Emergency Department

- Place the patient in a semireclining or full upright position
- Secure the airway and administer high-concentration oxygen
- Reassess the vital signs, including the respiratory and circulatory status

Prepare to administer the following drugs as appropriate, if not administered earlier:

- Administer a **nitroglycerin** 0.4-mg sublingual tablet or lingual aerosol and repeat every 5 min twice.

OR

Apply 1 to 1.5 inches of dermal nitroglycerin ointment.

AND/OR

Administer **morphine sulfate** 1 to 3 mg IV slowly and repeat every 5 to 30 min up to a total dose of 25 to 30 mg.

- Administer the following drugs:
  - ◇ **Furosemide** 40 to 80 mg IV slowly
  - ◇ **Digoxin** 0.5 mg IV over 5 min

If patient is in respiratory distress:

- Administer **aminophylline** 250 to 500 mg IV slowly over 20 to 30 min

If the patient is apprehensive/anxious:

- Administer **diazepam** 5 to 15 mg IV or **morphine sulfate** 1 to 3 mg IV slowly, if not administered earlier.

If nitroglycerin as administered above and morphine sulfate are not effective:

- Administer a nitroglycerin 12.5- to 25.0-μg IV bolus, followed by an IV infusion at a rate of 10 to 20 μg/min initially, then increasing the rate by 5 to 10 μg/min every 5 to 10 min if necessary as in step 3, *Adjunctive Treatment* in section B, *Initial Treatment and Assessment of Suspected Acute Myocardial Infarction*

Right Heart Failure Secondary to Right Ventricular Myocardial Infarction

Prehospital and/or Emergency Department as Appropriate

- Administer a **normal saline** 250- to 500-mL IV bolus rapidly; and repeat up to a total of 1 to 2 L or until the systolic blood pressure increases to 90 mm Hg or more.

If saline administration is ineffective:

- Administer **dobutamine** 2 to 20 μg/kg/min IV to increase and maintain the systolic blood pressure within normal limits.

E. MANAGEMENT OF CARDIOGENIC SHOCK
Prehospital/Emergency Department

- Place the patient in a face-up position, with legs elevated if pulmonary congestion and edema absent.
- Secure the airway and administer high-concentration oxygen.
- Reassess the vital signs, including the respiratory and circulatory status.

If the systolic blood pressure is less than 70 mm Hg initially:

- Administer a **norepinephrine** IV infusion at a rate of 0.5 to 1.0 μg/min initially and increase up to 8 to 30 μg/min to elevate the systolic blood pressure to 70 to 100 mm Hg.

OR

If the systolic blood pressure is 70 to 100 mm Hg initially:

- Administer a **dopamine** IV infusion at a rate of 2.5 to 5.0 μg/kg/min initially and increase up to 20 μg/kg/min to elevate and maintain the systolic blood pressure within normal limits.

If the shock condition continues for 1 hour in spite of maximum therapy, proceed with the following:

- Intraaortic balloon counterpulsation.

Caution!

Administer nitroglycerin and morphine sulfate with caution to patients with possible right ventricular MI while monitoring their pulse and blood pressure.

In addition, the level of consciousness and respiratory status must also be monitored in *all* patients receiving morphine sulfate, diazepam, and/or promethazine hydrochloride.

Caution!

β-blockers are contraindicated:

♦ If bradycardia (heart rate <60 bpm) is present
♦ If hypotension (systolic blood pressure <100 mm Hg) is present
♦ If PR interval >0.24 second or second- or third-degree AV block is present
♦ If congestive heart failure (left and/or right heart failure) is present
♦ If bronchospasm or a history of asthma is present
♦ If severe chronic obstructive pulmonary disease (COPD) is present, or
♦ If intravenous calcium channel blockers have been administered within a few hours

The patient's blood pressure and pulse must be monitored frequently during and after the administration of a β-blocker.

If hypotension occurs with a β-blocker, place the patient in a Trendelenburg position and administer a vasopressor.

If bradycardia, AV block, or asystole occurs, refer to the appropriate treatment protocol.

CONTRAINDICATIONS AND CAUTIONS FOR THE USE OF THROMBOLYTIC AGENTS IN ACUTE MYOCARDIAL INFARCTION

Absolute Contraindications

- Active internal bleeding (e.g., gastrointestinal or genitourinary)
- Previous hemorrhagic stroke at any time; other strokes or cerebrovascular events within the past year
- Recent intracranial or intraspinal surgery or trauma
- Known intracranial neoplasm, arteriovenous malformation, or cerebral aneurysm
- Severe uncontrolled hypertension during initial treatment and assessment ($\geq$180/110 mm Hg)
- Suspected aortic dissection

Cautions/Relative Contraindications

- Recent (within 2-4 weeks) major surgery (e.g., coronary artery bypass graft), obstetrical delivery, or organ biopsy
- Recent (within 2-4 weeks) trauma, including head trauma and cardiopulmonary resuscitation
- Previous puncture of noncompressible blood vessels
- Any other condition in which bleeding constitutes a significant hazard or would be particularly difficult to manage because of its location
- Known bleeding diathesis
- Current use of oral anticoagulants (e.g., warfarin sodium) with INR $\geq$2-3
- Diabetic hemorrhagic retinopathy or other hemorrhagic ophthalmic conditions
- History of recent (within 2-4 weeks) gastrointestinal, genitourinary, or other internal bleeding
- Active peptic ulcer
- Hemostatic defects including those secondary to severe hepatic or renal disease
- History of chronic hypertension ($\geq$180/110 mm Hg)
- History of prior cerebrovascular accident (CVA), seizures, or cerebrovascular disease not covered in *Absolute Contraindications* above
- High likelihood of left heart thrombus if mitral stenosis with atrial fibrillation is present without anticoagulation
- Subacute bacterial endocarditis
- Acute pericarditis
- Aortic aneurysm
- Septic thrombophlebitis or occluded AV cannula at a seriously infected site
- Severe hepatic or renal dysfunction
- Pregnancy or menstrual bleeding
- Advanced age
- Cancer or other terminal disease

PHASES OF THROMBUS FORMATION

Formation of a coronary artery thrombus consists of four phases: (1) platelet adhesion, (2) platelet activation, (3) platelet aggregation, and (4) thrombus formation.

Phase 1: Platelet Adhesion. At the moment an atherosclerotic plaque becomes denuded or ruptures, the platelets are exposed to collagen fibers and von Willebrand factor present within the cap of the atherosclerotic plaque. The platelets' GP Ia receptors bind with the collagen fibers; GP Ib and GP IIb/IIIa receptors bind with von Willebrand factor, which in turn also binds with the collagen fibers. The result is the adhesion of platelets to the collagen fibers within the plaque, forming a layer of platelets overlying the damaged plaque.

Phase 2: Platelet Activation. After being bound to the collagen fibers, the platelets become activated. The platelets change their shape from smooth ovals to tiny spheres while releasing adenosine diphosphate (ADP), serotonin, and thromboxane A_2 (TxA_2), substances that stimulate platelet aggregation. Platelet activation is also stimulated by the lipid-rich gruel within the atherosclerotic plaque. At the same time the GP IIb/IIIa receptors are turned on to bind with fibrinogen. While this is going on, tissue factor is being released from the tissue and platelets.

Phase 3: Platelet Aggregation. Once activated, the platelets bind to each other by means of fibrinogen, a cordlike structure that binds to the platelets' GP IIb/IIIa receptors. One fibrinogen can bind to two platelets, one at each end. Stimulated by ADP and TxA_2, the binding of fibrinogen to the GP IIb/IIIa receptors is greatly enhanced, resulting in a rapid growth of the platelet plug. By this time, the prothrombin has been converted to thrombin by the tissue factor.

Phase 4: Thrombus Formation. At first the platelet plug is rather unstable but becomes firmer as the fibrinogen between the platelets is replaced by stronger strands of fibrin. This occurs after prothrombin is converted to thrombin by tissue factor. Thrombin in turn converts fibrinogen to fibrin threads. Plasminogen usually becomes attached to the fibrin during its formation. As the thrombus grows, red cells and leucocytes (white cells) become entrapped in the platelet-fibrin mesh.

PHASES OF THROMBOLYSIS

Normally, the breakdown of a thrombus—*thrombolysis*—occurs when the thrombus is no longer needed to maintain the integrity of the blood vessel wall. Thrombolysis can also be initiated by the intravenous injection of thrombolytic agents such as alteplase, reteplase, and tenecteplase. Thrombolysis consists of three phases: (1) release of tissue plasminogen activator (tPA), (2) plasmin formation, and (3) fibrinolysis.

Phase 1: Release of tPA: Tissue plasminogen activator (tPA) is released from the endothelium of the blood vessel wall into the plasma.

Phase 2: Plasmin Formation. The tPA activates plasminogen attached to the fibrin strands within the thrombus, resulting in its conversion to plasmin.

Phase 3: Fibrinolysis. Plasmin breaks down the fibrin into soluble fragments causing the platelets to separate from each other and the thrombus to break apart.

Anti-Thrombus Drugs Used in the Management of Acute MI

Drug Category	Action	Drug
Antiplatelet agent	Inhibits thromboxane A_2 (TxA_2) formation and release from platelets, thereby inhibiting platelet aggregation	Aspirin
Anticoagulant	Blocks conversion of fibrinogen to fibrin by inhibiting the action of thrombin on fibrinogen	Low-molecular-weight-heparin: enoxaparin (Lovenox) Unfractionated heparin
GP IIb/IIIa receptor inhibitor	Inhibits platelet adhesion and aggregation by blocking the platelets' GP IIb/IIIa receptors	Abciximab (ReoPro) Eptifibatide (Integrilin)
Thrombolytic agent	Converts plasminogen to plasmin, which in turn dissolves the fibrin binding the platelets together	Alteplase (Activase) (t-PA) Reteplase (Retavase) (r-PA) Tenecteplase (TNKase) (TNK-tPA)

CHECKLIST TO DETERMINE A PATIENT'S ELIGIBILITY FOR THROMBOLYTIC THERAPY

Initial Patient Assessment

Yes No

- ☐ ☐ Patient oriented, cooperative, and reliable
- ☐ ☐ Age between 30 and 74 years
- ☐ ☐ Pain typical of acute MI
- ☐ ☐ Pain onset between 30 minutes and 6 hours at time of patient assessment
- ☐ ☐ Continuation of pain after administration of nitroglycerin
- ☐ ☐ History of previous MI
- ☐ ☐ Hypertension: systolic BP >180 mm Hg and/or diastolic BP >110 mm Hg
- ☐ ☐ Current use of warfarin (Coumadin) (i.e., "blood thinners") INR _____
- ☐ ☐ 12-lead ECG with significant ST segment and T wave changes
       Estimated time of arrival at ED _____

History

Yes No

- ☐ ☐ Recent (within 2 to 4 weeks) major surgery (e.g., intracranial or intraspinal surgery), obstetrical delivery, organ biopsy, or previous puncture of noncompressible blood vessels
- ☐ ☐ Recent (within 2 to 4 weeks) active internal bleeding (e.g., gastrointestinal or genitourinary bleeding)
- ☐ ☐ Recent (within 2 to 4 weeks) trauma (e.g., intracranial or intraspinal trauma) or cardiopulmonary resuscitation
- ☐ ☐ Pregnancy or active menstrual bleeding
- ☐ ☐ Hemostatic defects, including those secondary to severe hepatic or renal disease
- ☐ ☐ Known bleeding diathesis
- ☐ ☐ Significant hepatic dysfunction
- ☐ ☐ Diabetic hemorrhagic retinopathy, or other hemorrhagic ophthalmic conditions
- ☐ ☐ Any other condition in which bleeding may occur, especially if its management would be particularly difficult because of its location
- ☐ ☐ Severe uncontrollable hypertension
- ☐ ☐ Cerebrovascular disease, including cerebrovascular accident (CVA), seizures, cerebral aneurysm, intracranial neoplasm, or arteriovenous (AV) malformation
- ☐ ☐ Suspected aortic dissection or known aneurysm
- ☐ ☐ Suspected left heart thrombus secondary to atrial fibrillation associated with mitral stenosis
- ☐ ☐ Subacute bacterial endocarditis, septic thrombophlebitis, or an occluded AV cannula at a seriously infected site
- ☐ ☐ Pericarditis
- ☐ ☐ Cancer or other terminal disease

Appendix

Electrical conduction system

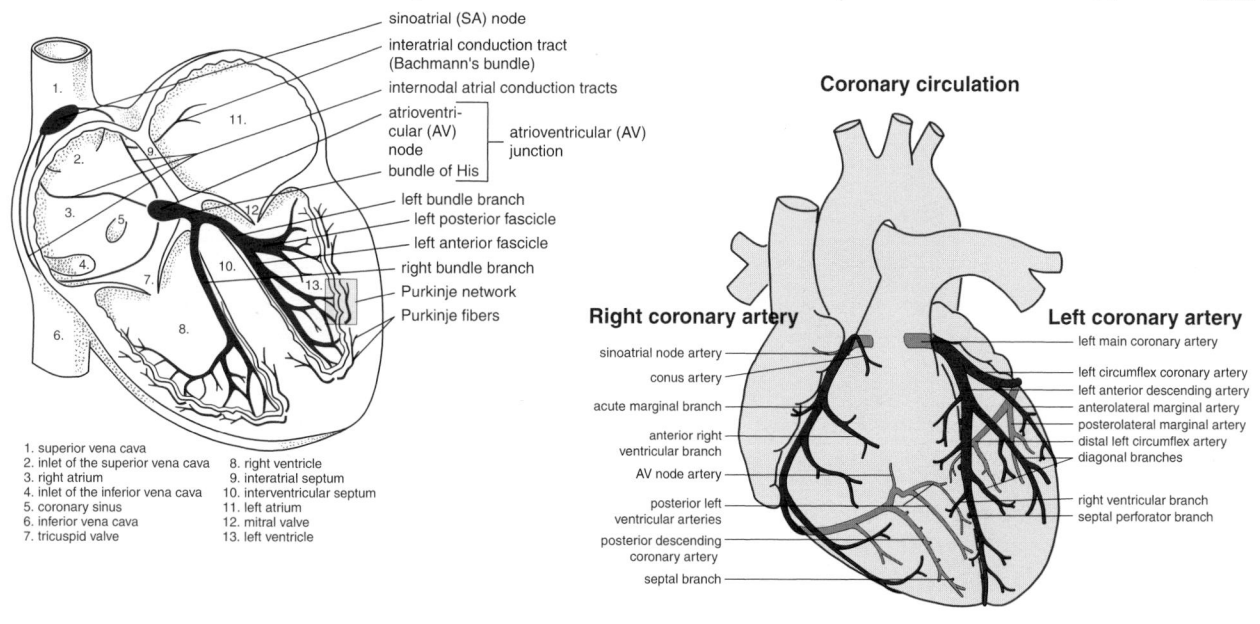

sinoatrial (SA) node

interatrial conduction tract
(Bachmann's bundle)

internodal atrial conduction tracts

atrioventri-
cular (AV)
node

atrioventricular (AV)
junction

bundle of His

left bundle branch
left posterior fascicle
left anterior fascicle
right bundle branch
Purkinje network
Purkinje fibers

1. superior vena cava
2. inlet of the superior vena cava
3. right atrium
4. inlet of the inferior vena cava
5. coronary sinus
6. inferior vena cava
7. tricuspid valve

8. right ventricle
9. interatrial septum
10. interventricular septum
11. left atrium
12. mitral valve
13. left ventricle

Coronary circulation

Right coronary artery

Left coronary artery

sinoatrial node artery
conus artery

acute marginal branch

anterior right
ventricular branch

AV node artery

posterior left
ventricular arteries

posterior descending
coronary artery

septal branch

left main coronary artery

left circumflex coronary artery
left anterior descending artery
anterolateral marginal artery
posterolateral marginal artery
distal left circumflex artery
diagonal branches

right ventricular branch
septal perforator branch

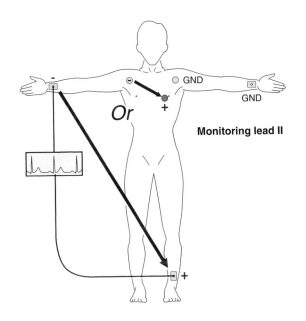

Monitoring lead II

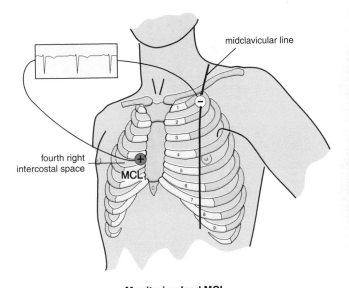

midclavicular line

fourth right
intercostal space

MCL

Monitoring lead MCL₁

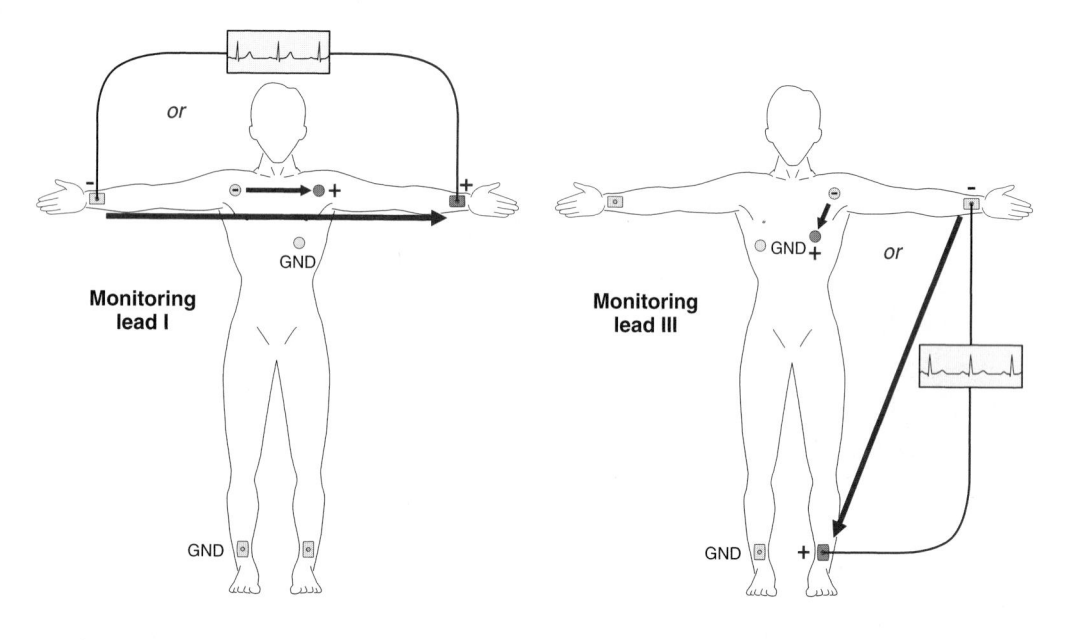

Monitoring lead I

Monitoring lead III

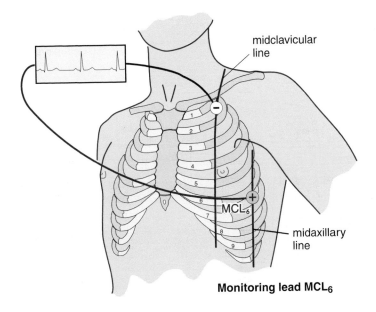

midclavicular line

midaxillary line

MCL$_6$

Monitoring lead MCL$_6$

The 12-Lead ECG

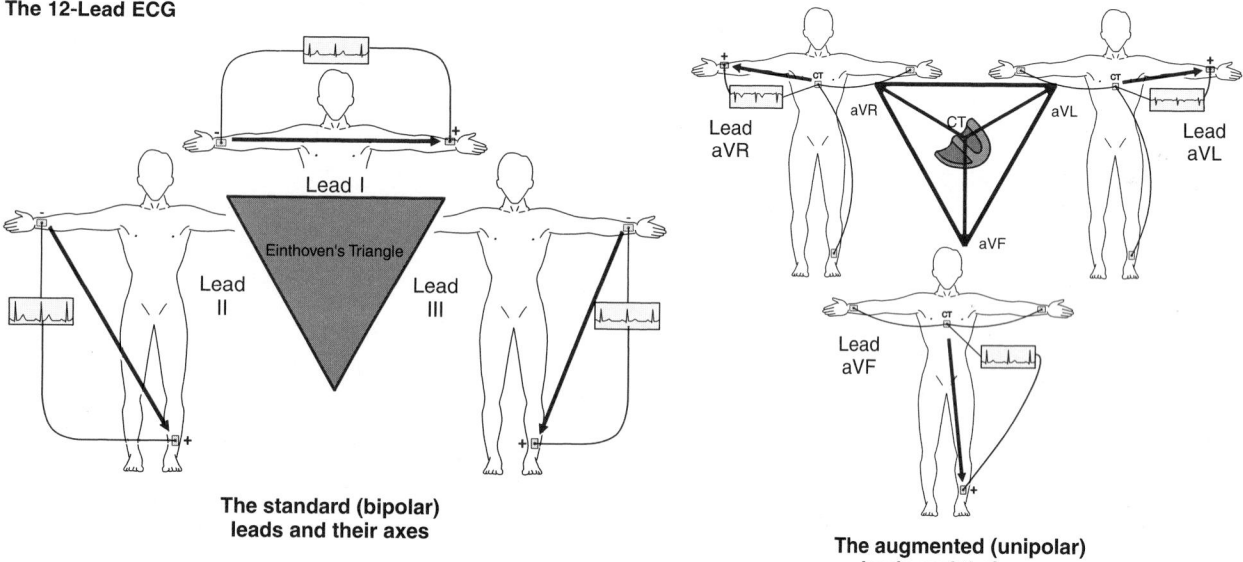

Einthoven's Triangle

Lead I

Lead II

Lead III

The standard (bipolar) leads and their axes

Lead aVR

Lead aVL

Lead aVF

aVR

aVL

aVF

CT

The augmented (unipolar) leads and their axes

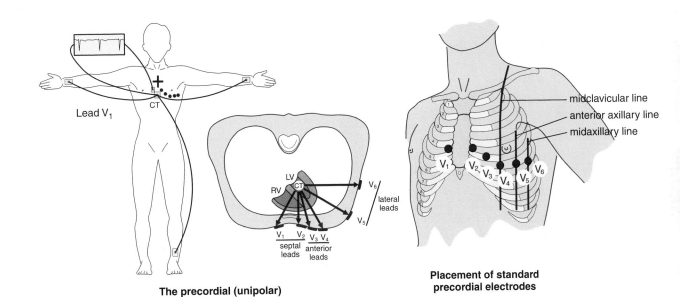

Lead V₁

LV
RV
CT

V₆
lateral
leads

V₅

V₁ V₂ V₃ V₄
septal   anterior
leads   leads

**The precordial (unipolar)
leads and their axes**

midclavicular line
anterior axillary line
midaxillary line

V₁ V₂ V₃ V₄ V₅ V₆

**Placement of standard
precordial electrodes**

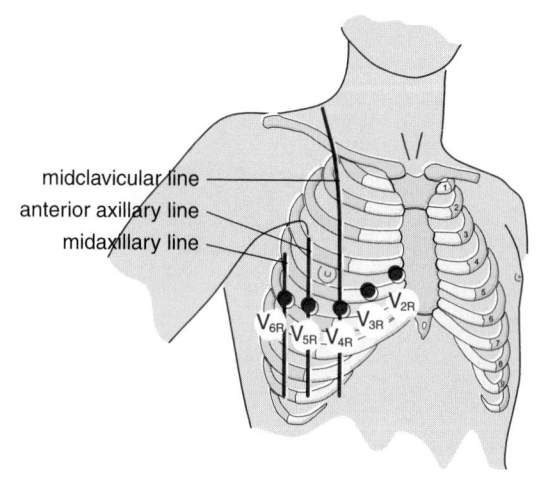

midclavicular line

anterior axillary line

midaxillary line

**Placement of right-sided
chest leads**

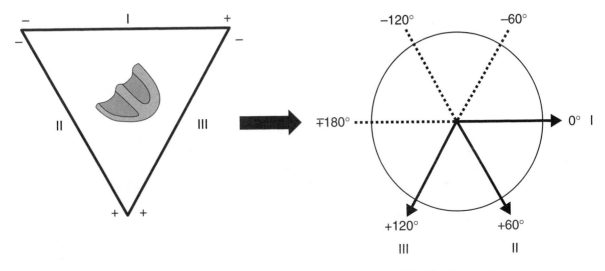

Einthoven's equilateral triangle
based on leads I, II, and III

Triaxial reference figure
for leads I, II, and III

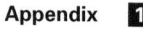

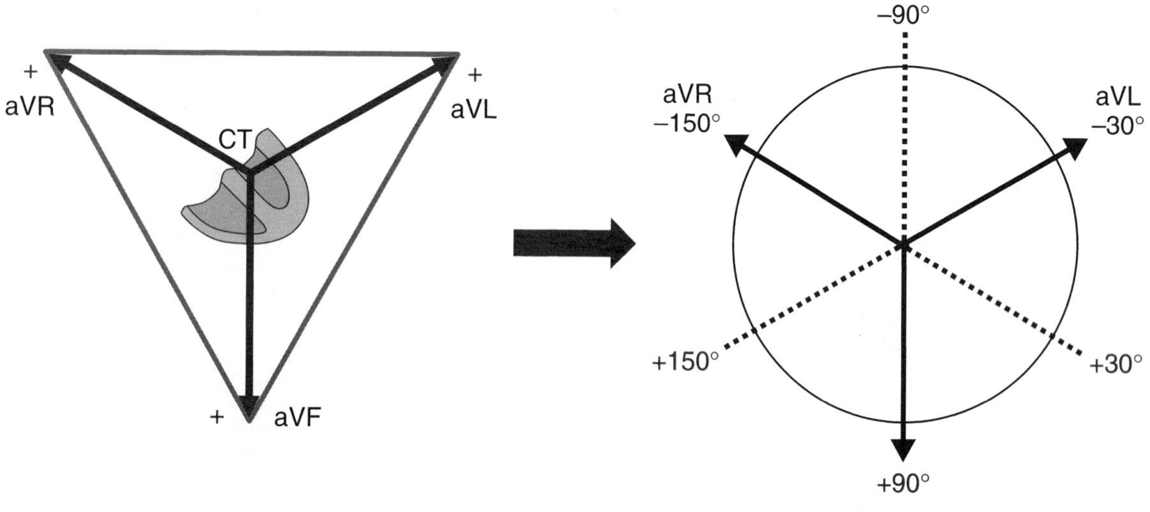

Triaxial reference figure for augmented leads aVR, aVL, and aVF

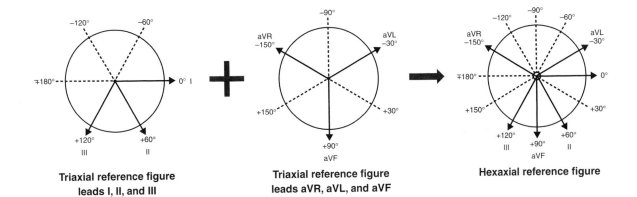

Triaxial reference figure leads I, II, and III

Triaxial reference figure leads aVR, aVL, and aVF

Hexaxial reference figure

THE THREE-LEAD METHOD OF DETERMINING THE QRS AXIS

If lead I is positive and:

A. Leads aVF and II are predominantly positive, the QRS axis is between 0° and +90°.

B. Lead aVF is predominantly negative, and lead II, predominantly positive, the QRS axis is between 0° and −30°.

C. Lead aVF is predominantly negative, and lead II, equiphasic, the QRS axis is exactly −30°.

D. Leads aVF and II are predominantly negative, the QRS axis is between −30° and −90°.

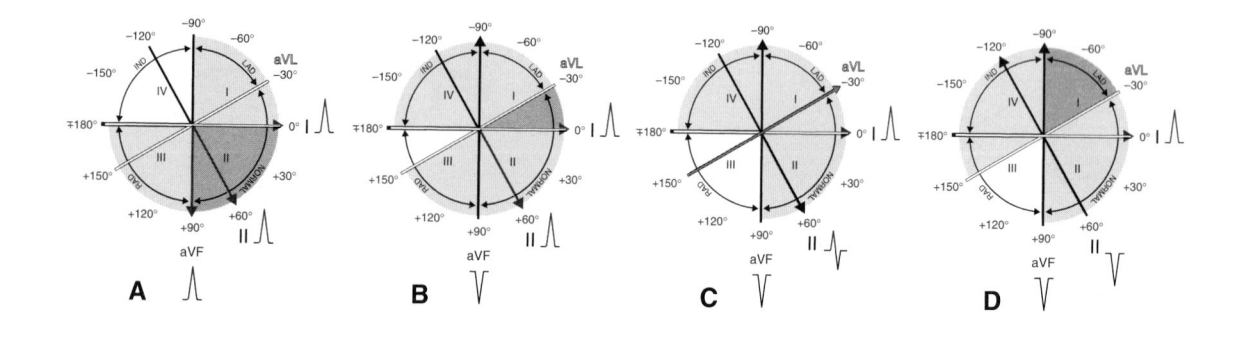

If lead I is negative and:

E(1). Leads aVF and II are predominantly positive, the QRS axis is between +90° and +150°.

E(2). If, in addition, lead aVR is also predominantly positive, the QRS axis is between +120° and +150°

F. Lead aVF is predominantly positive, and lead II, equiphasic, the QRS axis is exactly +150°.

G. Leads aVF and II are predominantly negative, the QRS axis is between −90° and −180°.

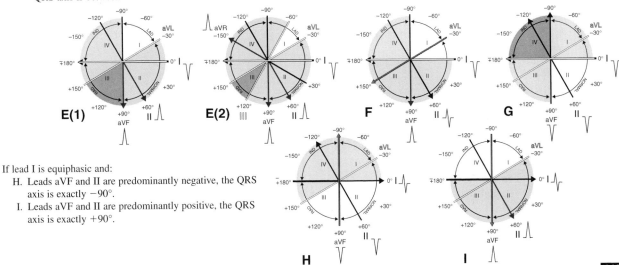

If lead I is equiphasic and:

H. Leads aVF and II are predominantly negative, the QRS axis is exactly −90°.

I. Leads aVF and II are predominantly positive, the QRS axis is exactly +90°.

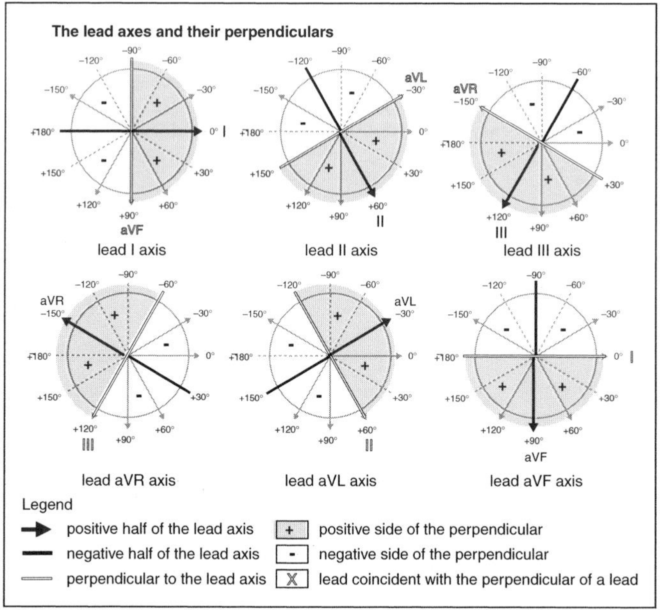

The lead axes and their perpendiculars

lead I axis

lead II axis

lead III axis

lead aVR axis

lead aVL axis

lead aVF axis

Legend

➡ positive half of the lead axis

▬ negative half of the lead axis

═ perpendicular to the lead axis

+ positive side of the perpendicular

- negative side of the perpendicular

X lead coincident with the perpendicular of a lead

Normal and Abnormal QRS axes

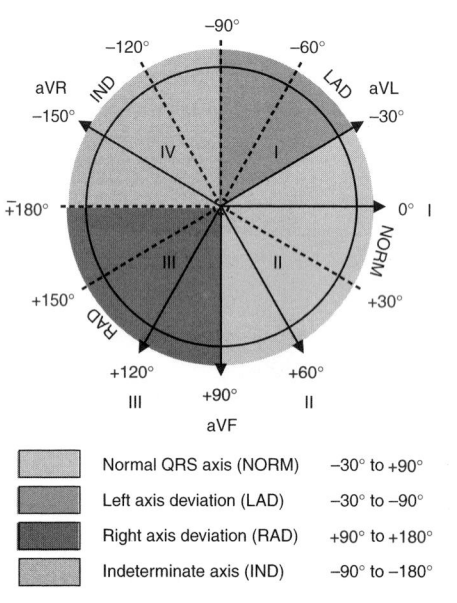

Normal QRS axis (NORM)	−30° to +90°
Left axis deviation (LAD)	−30° to −90°
Right axis deviation (RAD)	+90° to +180°
Indeterminate axis (IND)	−90° to −180°

COMPONENTS OF THE ELECTROCARDIOGRAM

Waves

P wave
  Normal sinus P wave
  Abnormal sinus P wave
  Ectopic P wave (P prime or P′)
QRS complex
  Normal QRS complex
  Abnormal QRS complex
T wave
  Normal T wave
  Abnormal T wave
U wave

Intervals

PR interval
  Normal PR interval
  Abnormal PR interval
QT interval
  Normal QT interval
  Abnormal QT interval
R-R interval

Segments

ST segment
  Normal ST segment
  Abnormal ST segment
PR segment
TP segment

WAVES

P Wave

Normal Sinus P Wave

Significance: Represents normal depolarization of the right and left atria, which proceeds from right to left and downward.
Pacemaker Site: SA node.

ECG Characteristics

Direction: Positive (upright) in lead II.
Duration: 0.10 second or less.
Amplitude: 0.5 to 2.5 mm in lead II.
Shape: Smooth and rounded.
P Wave-QRS Complex Relationship: Each normally followed by a QRS complex; exception: AV block.
PR Interval: May be normal (0.12 to 0.20 second) or abnormal (greater than 0.20 second or less than 0.12 second).

Abnormal Sinus P Wave

Significance: Represents depolarization of altered, damaged, or abnormal atria, which

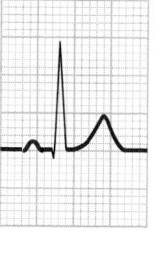

II

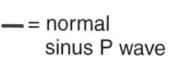

— = normal
sinus P wave

proceeds from right to left and downward. Abnormal sinus P waves may be seen in the following:

- Increased right atrial pressure and right atrial dilatation and hypertrophy (right atrial overload) resulting from chronic obstructive pulmonary disease (COPD), status asthmaticus, acute pulmonary embolism, and acute pulmonary edema (tall and symmetrically peaked P waves **[P pulmonale]** in leads II, III, and aVF; biphasic P waves in leads V_1-V_2)
- Sinus tachycardia (abnormally tall P waves)
- Increased left atrial pressure and left atrial dilatation and hypertrophy (left atrial overload) resulting from hypertension, mitral and aortic valvular disease, acute MI, and pulmonary edema secondary to left heart failure (wide, notched P waves **[P mitrale]** in leads I, II, and V_4-V_6; biphasic P waves in lead V_1)
- Delay or block of the progression of electrical impulses through the interatrial conduction tract between the right and left atria (wide, notched P waves **[P mitrale]**)

Pacemaker Site: SA node.

ECG Characteristics

Direction: Positive (upright) in lead II.

Duration: May be normal (0.10 second or less) or greater than 0.10 second.

Amplitude: May be normal (0.5 to 2.5 mm) or greater than 2.5 mm in lead II. A P pulmonale is 2.5 mm or greater in amplitude.

Shape: May be tall and symmetrically peaked *(P pulmonale)* or wide and notched *(P mitrale)* in lead II and biphasic in leads V_1 and V_2.

P Wave-QRS Complex Relationship: Each normally followed by a QRS complex; exception: AV block.

PR Interval: May be normal (0.12 to 0.20 second) or abnormal (greater than 0.20 second or less than 0.12 second).

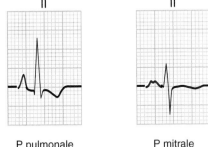

— = abnormal sinus P wave   P pulmonale   P mitrale

Ectopic P Wave (P Prime or P′)

Significance: Represents abnormal atrial depolarization occurring in an abnormal direction or sequence or both, the direction and sequence depending on the ectopic pacemaker's location.

- If the ectopic pacemaker is in the upper or middle part of the right atrium, depolarization of the atria occurs in a normal direction (right to left and downward).
- If the ectopic pacemaker is in the lower part of the right atrium near the AV node or in the left atrium or if it is in the AV junction or the ventricles, in which case the electrical impulse travels upward through the AV junction into the atria (retrograde conduction), the atria depolarize from left to right and upward (retrograde atrial depolarization).

Ectopic P waves occur in various atrial, junctional, and ventricular arrhythmias, including the following:

- Wandering atrial pacemaker
- Premature atrial contractions
- Atrial tachycardia
- Premature junctional contractions
- Junctional escape rhythm
- Nonparoxysmal junctional tachycardia
- Paroxysmal supraventricular tachycardia
- Premature ventricular contractions (occasionally)

Pacemaker Site: An ectopic pacemaker in the atria outside of the SA node or in the AV junction or ventricles.

ECG Characteristics

Direction

- Positive (upright) in lead II, often resembling a normal sinus P wave, if the ectopic pacemaker is in the upper or middle right atrium
- Negative (inverted) in lead II if the ectopic pacemaker is in the lower right atrium near the AV node or in the left atrium, AV junction, or ventricles

Duration: 0.10 second or less or greater then 0.10 second.

Amplitude: Usually less than 2.5 mm in lead II, but may be greater.

Shape: May be smooth and rounded, peaked, or slightly notched.

P Wave-QRS Complex Relationship: May precede, be buried in, or follow the QRS complex with which it is associated.

P′R/RP′ Interval: Relationship between site of ectopic pacemaker, type of interval, and duration:

- Upper or middle part of the right atrium: P′R interval normal (0.12 to 0.20 second) *(A)*
- Lower part of the atria, close to the AV node: P′R interval slightly less than 0.12 second *(B)*
- Upper part of the AV junction: P′R interval less than 0.12 second *(C)*
- Lower part of the AV junction or in the ventricles: RP′ interval usually less than 0.20 second *(D)*

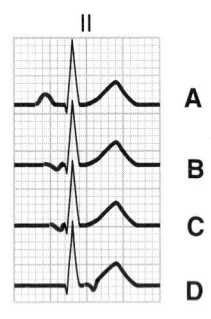

QRS Complex

Normal QRS Complex

Significance: Represents normal depolarization of the right and left ventricles, which begins with the depolarization of the interventricular septum from left to right producing the Q wave and then continues with the depolarization of the ventricles from the endocardium to the epicardium producing the R and S waves.

Pacemaker Site: The SA node or an ectopic or escape pacemaker in the atria or AV junction.

ECG Characteristics

Components: The QRS complex consists of one or more of the following positive (upright) deflections (the R waves) and negative (inverted) deflections (the Q, S, and QS waves):

♦ **R wave:** The first positive deflection in the QRS complex. Subsequent positive deflections that extend above the baseline are called *R prime (R′), R double prime (R″),* and so forth.

♦ **Q wave:** The first negative deflection in the QRS complex not preceded by an R wave.

♦ **S wave:** The first negative deflection that extends below the baseline in the QRS complex following an R wave. Subsequent negative deflections are called *S prime (S′), S double prime (S″),* and so forth.

♦ **QS wave:** A QRS complex that consists entirely of a single, large negative deflection.

NOTE: Although there may be only one Q wave, there can be more than one R and S wave in the QRS complex.

♦ **Notch:** A notch in the R wave is a negative deflection that does not extend below the baseline; a notch in the S wave is a positive deflection that does not extend above the baseline.

The large waves that form the major deflections are identified by upper case letters (**QS, R, S**). The smaller waves that are less than one-half the amplitude of the major deflections are identified by lower case letters (q, r, s). Thus the ventricular depolarization complex can be described more accurately by using upper and lower case letters assigned to the waves (e.g., **qR, Rs, qRs**).

Direction: May be predominantly positive (upright), predominantly negative (inverted), or equiphasic (equally positive, equally negative).

Duration

    QRS complex: 0.10 second or less (0.06 to 0.10) in adults and 0.08 second or less in children.

    Q wave: 0.04 second or less.

    Ventricular activation time (VAT): The time from the onset of the QRS complex to the peak of the R wave; normally 0.05 second or less, but may be greater than 0.05 second in left ventricular hypertrophy.

Amplitude: The amplitude of the R or S wave in the QRS complex in lead II may vary from 1 to 2 mm to 15 mm or more. The normal Q wave is less than 25% of the height of the succeeding R wave.

Shape: The QRS complex waves are generally narrow and sharply pointed.

Junction (J) Point: The end of the QRS complex at the point where the QRS complex becomes the ST segment.

II · II · III

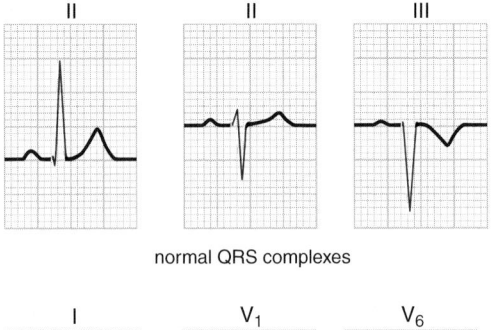

normal QRS complexes

**Normal and Abnormal
QRS Complexes**

V_1 · V_6

II · II

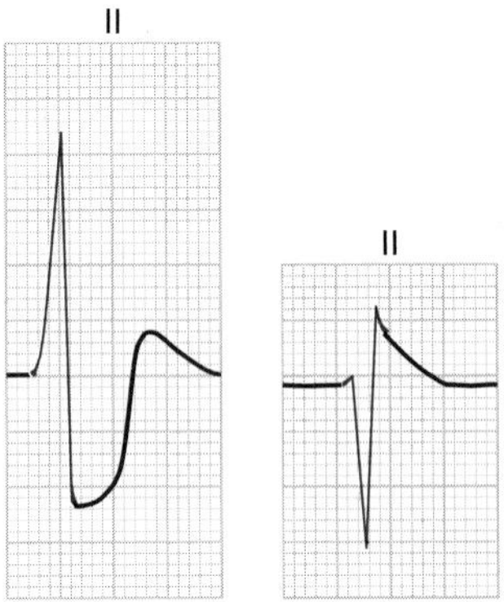

premature ventricular contractions

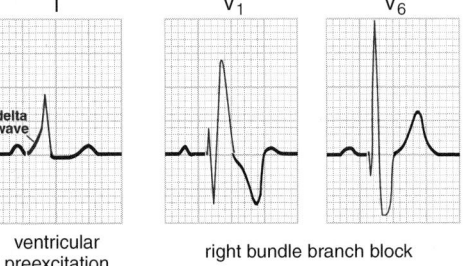

I · V_1 · V_6

delta
wave

ventricular
preexcitation · right bundle branch block

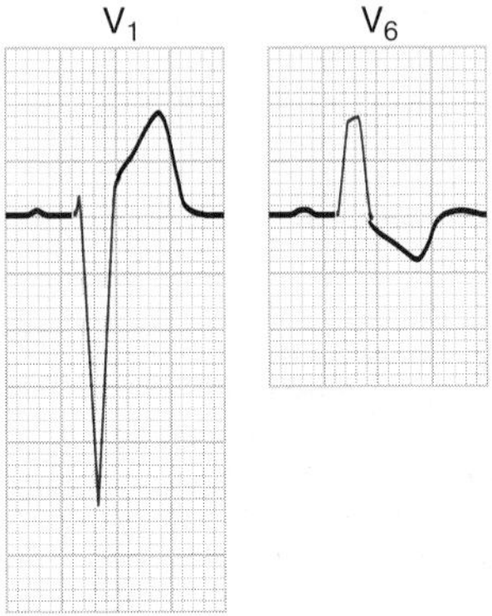

left bundle branch block

▬ = QRS complex

Abnormal QRS Complex

Significance: Represents abnormal depolarization of the ventricles, which may result from one of the following:

- **Intraventricular conduction disturbance.** The most common forms are right and left bundle branch block; a less common form, a nonspecific, diffuse intraventricular conduction defect (IVCD), is seen in myocardial infarction, fibrosis, and hypertrophy; electrolyte imbalance, such as hypokalemia and hyperkalemia; and excessive administration of such cardiac drugs as quinidine, procainamide, and flecainide. May be seen in supraventricular rhythms and arrhythmias.

- **Aberrant ventricular conduction (aberrancy).** A temporary delay in the conduction of an electrical impulse through the bundle branches usually caused by the appearance of the electrical impulse at the bundle branches prematurely while they are still partially refractory and unable to conduct normally. The result is an abnormally wide QRS complex that often resembles an incomplete or complete bundle branch block. Aberrancy is most commonly seen in premature atrial and junctional contractions and supraventricular tachyarrhythmias.

- **Ventricular preexcitation.** Premature depolarization of the ventricles caused by abnormal conduction of electrical impulses from the atria or AV junction to the ventricles via an accessory conduction pathway (the *accessory AV pathway*) bypassing the AV junction—the classic form of ventricular preexcitation. The result is a shorter than normal PR interval (0.09 to 0.12 sec) and a wide QRS complex (0.10 sec or more) with an initial slurring of the upward slope of the R wave (or of the downstroke of the S wave, as the case may be)—the *delta wave.* Another preexcitation syndrome, the *nodoventricular/fasciculoventricular preexcitation,* involving an accessory conduction pathway between the lower part of the AV node or the bundle of His and the ventricles (the nodoventricular/fasciculoventricular fibers), also results in an abnormally wide QRS complex with a delta wave but with a normal PR interval. May be seen in supraventricular rhythms and arrhythmias.

- **Ventricular arrhythmias.** Arrhythmias that originate in a ventricular ectopic or escape pacemaker located in the bundle branches, Purkinje network, or ventricular myocardium.

Pacemaker site: The SA node or an ectopic or escape pacemaker in the atria, AV junction, or ventricles.

ECG Characteristics

Components: The same as in normal QRS complexes. In addition, if ventricular preexcitation is present, an initial delta wave is usually present.

Direction: May be predominantly positive (upright), predominantly negative (inverted), or equiphasic (equally positive, equally negative).

Duration: Greater than 0.10 second.
Amplitude: Varies from 1 to 2 mm to 20 mm or more.
Shape: Varies widely in shape, from one that appears quite normal—narrow and sharply pointed (as in incomplete bundle branch block and aberrant ventricular conduction and in ventricular arrhythmias arising in the bundle branches)—to one that is wide and bizarre, slurred and notched (as in complete bundle branch block and aberrant ventricular conduction and in ventricular arrhythmias arising in the Purkinje network and ventricular myocardium).

T Wave

Normal T Wave
Significance: Represents normal repolarization of the ventricles, which proceeds from the epicardium to the endocardium.
ECG Characteristics
Direction: Positive (upright) in lead II.

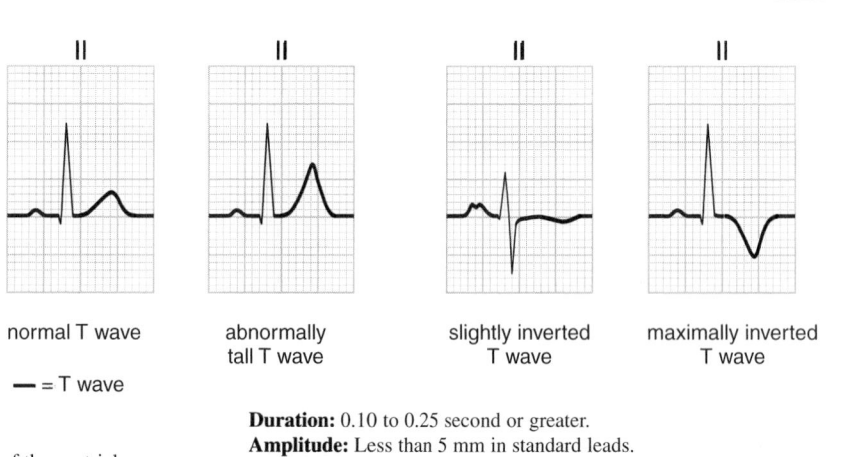

normal T wave

— = T wave

abnormally tall T wave

slightly inverted T wave

maximally inverted T wave

Duration: 0.10 to 0.25 second or greater.
Amplitude: Less than 5 mm in standard leads.
Shape: Sharply or bluntly rounded and slightly asymmetrical, the first, upward part being longer than the second, downward part.
T Wave-QRS Complex Relationship: Always follows the QRS complex.

Abnormal T Wave

Significance: Represents abnormal ventricular repolarization, which may proceed (a) from the epicardium to the endocardium as it normally does, but at a slower rate than usual, producing an abnormally tall, upright T wave in lead II, or (b) from the endocardium to the epicardium, producing a negative T wave in lead II. Abnormal ventricular repolarization may occur in the following:

- Myocardial ischemia associated with ACS, myocarditis, pericarditis
- Ventricular enlargement (hypertrophy)
- Electrolyte imbalance (e.g., excess serum potassium)
- Administration of certain cardiac drugs (e.g., quinidine, procainamide)
- Bundle branch block and ectopic ventricular arrhythmias
- In athletes and in persons who are hyperventilating

ECG Characteristics

Direction: May be positive (upright) and abnormally tall or low, negative (inverted), or biphasic (partially positive and partially negative) in lead II. The abnormal T wave may or may not be in the same direction as that of the normal QRS complex. The T wave following an abnormal QRS complex is almost always opposite in direction to it and abnormally wide and tall or deeply inverted.

Duration: 0.10 to 0.25 second or greater.

Amplitude: Variable.

Shape: May be rounded, blunt, sharply peaked, wide, or notched.

U Wave

Significance: Probably represents the final stage of repolarization of a small segment of the ventricles (such as the papillary muscles or ventricular septum) after most of the right and left ventricles have been repolarized. Abnormally tall U waves may be present in the following:

♦ Hypokalemia
♦ Cardiomyopathy, left ventricular hypertrophy
♦ Excessive administration of digitalis, quinidine, procainamide, and amiodarone

ECG Characteristics

Location: On the downward slope of the T wave or following it.
Direction: Normally positive (upright), the same direction as that of the preceding normal T wave in lead II. Abnormal U waves may be positive (upright) or negative (inverted).
Duration: Usually not determined.
Amplitude: Normally less than 2 mm and always smaller than that of the preceding T wave in lead II. A U wave taller than 2 mm or the preceding T wave is considered to be abnormal.
Shape: Rounded and symmetrical.

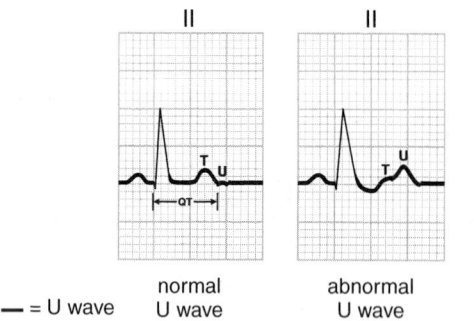

— = U wave

normal U wave

abnormal U wave

INTERVALS

QT Interval
Normal QT Interval

Significance: Represents the time between the onset of depolarization and the end of repolarization of the ventricles (i.e., the refractory period of the ventricles) and indicates that ventricular repolarization is normal.

ECG Characteristics

Onset and End: Begins with the onset of the QRS complex and ends with the end of the T wave.

Duration: Dependent on the heart rate, being shorter when the heart rate is fast and longer when the heart rate is slow. Normally, the QT interval is somewhat less then half of the preceding R-R interval, one that is greater than half is abnormal, and one that is about half is "borderline." The QT intervals may be equal or unequal in duration depending on the underlying rhythm. The average duration of the QT interval normally expected at a given heart rate, the *corrected QT interval* (or *QTc*), and the normal range of 10% above and 10% below the average value are shown in the table to the right. Regardless of the heart rate, a QT interval of greater than 0.45 second is considered abnormal.

NOTE: The determination of the QT interval should be made in the lead where the T wave is most prominent and not deformed by a U

QTc Intervals

Heart Rate/min	R-R Interval (sec)	QTc (sec) and Normal Range
40	1.5	0.46 (0.41-0.51)
50	1.2	0.42 (0.38-0.46)
60	1.0	0.39 (0.35-0.43)
70	0.86	0.37 (0.33-0.41)
80	0.75	0.35 (0.32-0.39)
90	0.67	0.33 (0.30-0.36)
100	0.60	0.31 (0.28-0.34)
120	0.50	0.29 (0.26-0.32)
150	0.40	0.25 (0.23-0.28)
180	0.33	0.23 (0.21-0.25)
200	0.30	0.22 (0.20-0.24)

wave and should not include the U wave. Furthermore, the measurement of the QT interval assumes that the duration of the QRS complex is normal with an average value of 0.08 second. If the QRS is widened beyond 0.08 second for any reason, the excess widening beyond 0.08 second must be subtracted from the actual measurement to obtain the correct QT interval.

Abnormal QT Interval

Significance: Represents an abnormal rate of ventricular repolarization, either slower or more rapid than normal. An abnormally prolonged QT interval, one that exceeds the average QT interval for any given heart rate by 10%, indicates slowing of ventricular repolarization. This can occur in the following:

◆ Electrolyte imbalance (hypokalemia and hypocalcemia)
◆ Excess of certain drugs (e.g., quinidine, procainamide, disopyramide, amiodarone, phenothiazines, and tricyclic antidepressants). The prolongation of the QT interval following administration of excessive amounts of such antiarrhythmic agents as quinidine, procainamide, and disopyramide, may provoke the appearance of torsade de pointes.
◆ Liquid protein diets
◆ Pericarditis, acute myocarditis, acute myocardial ischemia and infarction, and left ventricular hypertrophy
◆ Hypothermia
◆ Central nervous system disorders (e.g., cerebrovascular accident [CVA], subarachnoid hemorrhage, intracranial trauma)
◆ Without a known cause (idiopathic)
◆ Bradyarrhythmias (e.g., marked sinus bradycardia, third-degree AV block with slow ventricular escape rhythm)

An abnormally short QT interval, one that is less than the average QT interval (QTc) for any given heart rate by 10%, represents an increase in the rate of repolarization of the ventricles. This can occur in the following:

◆ Digitalis therapy
◆ Hypercalcemia

ECG Characteristics

Onset and End: The same as those of a normal PR interval.

Duration: Greater or less than the QTc for any given heart rate by 10%. A QT interval of greater than 0.45 second is considered abnormal regardless of the heart rate.

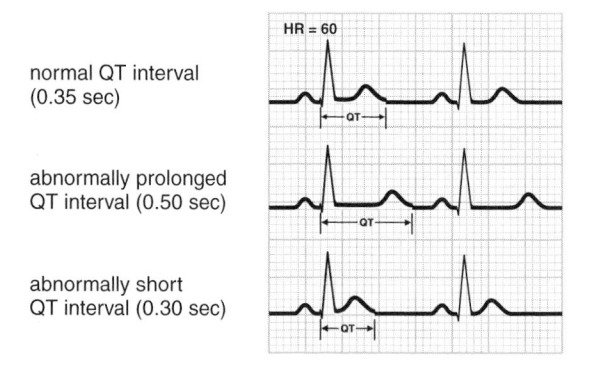

normal QT interval
(0.35 sec)

abnormally prolonged
QT interval (0.50 sec)

abnormally short
QT interval (0.30 sec)

R-R Interval

Significance: Represents the time between two successive ventricular depolarizations during which the atria and ventricles contract and relax once (i.e., one cardiac cycle).

ECG Characteristics

Onset and End: Begins with the peak of one R wave and ends with the peak of the succeeding R wave.

Duration: Dependent on the heart rate, being shorter when the heart rate is fast and longer when the heart rate is slow (e.g., heart rate 120, R-R interval 0.50 second; heart rate 60, R-R interval 1.0 second). The R-R intervals may be equal or unequal in duration depending on the underlying rhythm.

PR Interval
Normal PR Interval

Significance: Represents the time from the onset of atrial depolarization to the onset of ventricular depolarization during which the electrical impulse progresses normally and without delay from the SA node or an ectopic pacemaker in the atria near the SA node through the electrical conduction system to the ventricular myocardium. The PR interval includes the P wave and PR segment.

ECG Characteristics

Onset and End: Begins with the onset of the P wave and ends with the onset of the QRS complex.

Duration: Varies from 0.12 to 0.20 second, depending on the heart rate. Normally, it is shorter when the heart rate is fast and longer when the heart rate is slow (e.g., heart rate 120, PR interval 0.16 second; heart rate 60, PR interval 0.20 second).

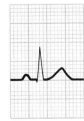

— = PR interval   normal PR interval

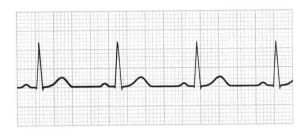

— = R-R interval

Abnormal PR Interval

Significance: Represents the abnormal progression of the electrical impulse from the SA node or an ectopic or escape supraventricular pacemaker through the electrical conduction system to the ventricular myocardium. It may be greater than 0.20 second or less than 0.12 second.

— = PR interval

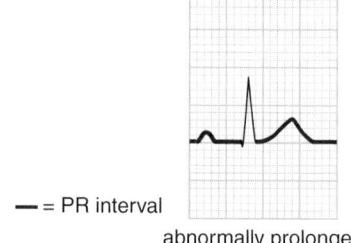

abnormally prolonged
PR interval

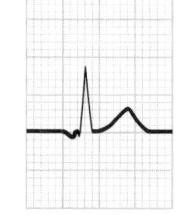
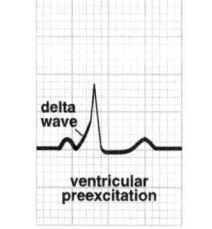
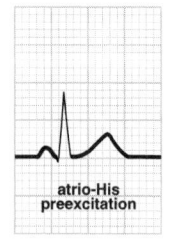

delta wave

ventricular
preexcitation

atrio-His
preexcitation

abnormally short PR interval

◆ When greater than 0.20 second, it represents delayed progression of the electrical impulse through the AV node, bundle of His, or, rarely, the bundle branches—AV block.

◆ When less than 0.12 second, it represents either:
(a) the origination of the electrical impulse in an ectopic pacemaker in the atria close to the AV node or in an ectopic or escape pacemaker in the AV junction; in both instances the P waves are commonly negative (inverted) in lead II

OR

(b) the abnormal progression of the electrical impulse from the atria to the ventricles through an accessory conduction pathway that either bypasses the AV junction via the accessory AV pathway *(ventricular preexcitation)* or the AV node alone via the atrio-His fibers *(atrio-His preexcitation)*. The P waves in these preexcitation syndromes are usually positive (upright) in lead II. The QRS complexes in ventricular preexcitation are abnormally wide, with a delta wave; those in atrio-His preexcitation are normal.

ECG Characteristics

Onset and End: The same as those of a normal PR interval.

Duration: May be greater than 0.20 second or less than 0.12 second.

SEGMENTS

ST Segment

Normal ST Segment
Significance: Represents the early part of normal repolarization of the right and left ventricles.

ECG Characteristics

Onset and End: Begins with the end of the QRS complex, the "Junction" or "J" point, and ends with the onset of the T wave.

Duration: 0.20 second or less, depending on the heart rate, being shorter when the heart rate is fast and longer when the heart rate is slow.

Amplitude: Normally flat (isoelectric), but may be slightly elevated or depressed by less than 1.0 mm, 0.04 second (1 small square) after the J point of the QRS complex and still be normal.

Appearance: If slightly elevated, may be flat, concave, or arched. If slightly depressed, may be flat, upsloping, or downsloping.

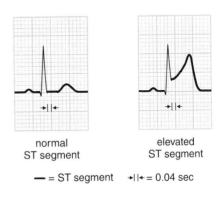

normal
ST segment

elevated
ST segment

━ = ST segment   ⇥||⇤ = 0.04 sec

Abnormal ST Segment

Significance: Represents the early part of abnormal repolarization of the right and left ventricles, a common consequence of myocardial ischemia and injury, and pericarditis. It is also present in ventricular fibrosis and aneurysm, left ventricular hypertrophy, and administration of digitalis. ST segment elevation may also occur normally as "early repolarization."

ECG Characteristics

Onset and End: Same as those of a normal ST segment.

Duration: 0.20 second or less, depending on the heart rate.

Amplitude: Elevated or depressed 1.0 mm or more, 0.04 second (1 small square) after the J point of the QRS complex.

Appearance: If elevated, may be flat, concave, or arched. If depressed, may be flat, upsloping, or downsloping.

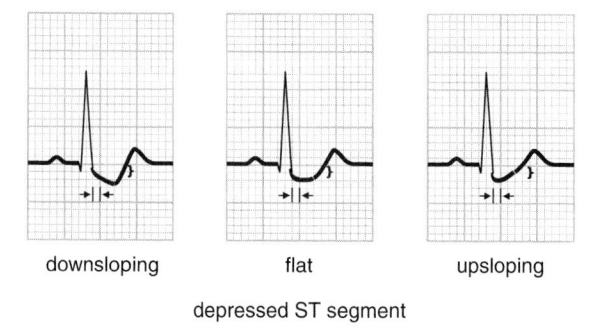

downsloping   flat   upsloping

depressed ST segment

— = ST segment →||← = 0.04 sec } = ST depression >1 m

PR Segment

Significance: Represents the time from the end of atrial depolarization to the onset of ventricular depolarization during which the electrical impulse progresses from the AV node through the bundle of His, bundle branches, and Purkinje network to the ventricular myocardium.

ECG Characteristics

Onset and End: Begins with the end of the P wave and ends with the onset of the QRS complex.

Duration: Normally varies from about 0.02 to 0.10 second, but may be greater than 0.10 second if there is a delay in the progression of the electrical impulse through the AV node, bundle of His, or, rarely, the bundle branches.

Amplitude: Normally, flat (isoelectric).

TP Segment

Significance: Represents the time from the end of ventricular repolarization to the onset of the following atrial depolarization—the interval between two successive P-QRS-T complexes, during which electrical activity of the heart is absent. It includes the U wave if one is present.

ECG Characteristics

Onset and End: Begins with the end of the T wave and ends with the onset of the following P wave.

Duration: 0.0 to 0.4 second or greater depending on the heart rate, being shorter when the heart rate is fast and longer when the heart rate is slow (e.g., heart rate about 120 or greater, TP segment 0 second: heart rate about 60 or less, TP segment 0.4 second or greater).

Amplitude: Usually flat (isoelectric).

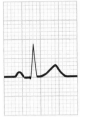

— = PR segment

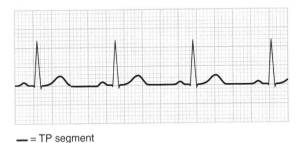

— = TP segment

NORMAL ECG COMPONENTS

P Waves: Normally, each followed by a QRS complex.

Direction: Positive (upright) in leads I, II, aVF, and V_4-V_6. Negative (inverted) in lead aVR. Positive, negative, or diphasic in leads III, aVL, and V_1-V_3.

Duration: 0.10 second or less.

Amplitude: 0.5 to 2.5 mm in lead II.

Shape: Smooth and rounded.

QRS Complexes: 0.10 second or less with generally narrow and sharply pointed waves.

Q waves: 0.04 second or less in duration and less than 25% of the height of the succeeding R wave.

Ventricular activation time (VAT): 0.05 second or less.

T Waves: Amplitude less than 5 mm in the standard limb and unipolar leads; less than 10 mm in the precordial leads.

PR Intervals: 0.12 to 0.20 second.

QT Intervals: Less than half the preceding R-R interval.

ST Segments: Flat, but may be elevated or depressed by no more than 1.0 mm, 0.04 second (1 small square) after the J point.

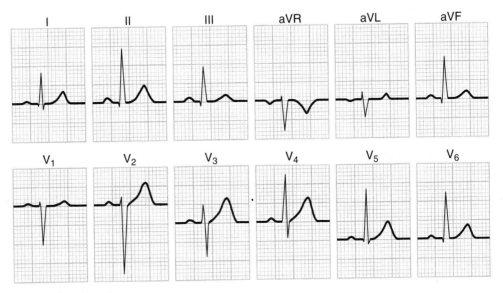

normal electrocardiogram

ECG INTERPRETATION

The following is an outline of the steps in interpreting an ECG to determine the presence of an arrhythmia and its identity. The ECG interpretation may be performed in the order shown or in accordance with local prehospital or hospital protocols.

Arrhythmia Determination

Step One: Determine the heart rate.

Step Two: Determine the ventricular rhythm.

Step Three: Identify and analyze the P, P', F, or f waves.
1. Identify the P, P', F, or f waves.
2. Determine the atrial rate and rhythm.
3. Note the relationship of the P, P', F, or f waves to the QRS complexes.

Step Four: Determine the PR or RP' intervals and AV conduction ratio.
1. Determine the PR (or RP') intervals.
2. Assess the equality of the PR (or RP') intervals.
3. Determine the AV conduction ratio.

Step Five: Identify and analyze the QRS complexes.
1. Identify the QRS complexes.
2. Note the duration and shape of the QRS complexes.
3. Assess the equality of the QRS complexes.

Step Six: Determine the site of origin of the arrhythmia.

Step Seven: Identify the arrhythmia.

Step Eight: Evaluate the significance of the arrhythmia.

The following is an outline of the steps in interpreting a 12-lead ECG to determine the presence of an acute MI, its location, and the estimated time of onset. The ECG interpretation may be performed in the order shown or in accordance with local prehospital or hospital protocols.

Acute Myocardial Infarction Determination

Step One: Identify any abnormally elevated or depressed ST segments and the leads where noted.

Step Two: Identify any abnormally tall or inverted T waves and the leads where noted.

Step Three: Identify any Q waves and the leads where noted.

Step Four: Identify any abnormally tall, diminished, or absent R waves and the leads where noted.

Step Five: Based on the above analysis, determine:
1. The presence or absence of an acute MI.
2. The location of the acute MI.
3. The estimated onset of the acute MI.

INDEX

Page numbers followed by f indicate figures; t, tables.